Quantitative Research for Chaplains and Health Care Professionals: A Primer

T0372918

This book takes readers from very basic research concepts, such as 'causality' and 'variables', to the application of different types of statistical analyses. The first two chapters introduce the scientific method and causality, and assess the degree to which the major types of research designs used in health care studies allow researchers to make causal inferences. The book concludes with a detailed description of the seven critical factors that must be controlled to draw causal inferences from experimental studies. The rest of the book covers levels of measurement, i.e. nominal, ordinal, interval, and ratio scales; operational definitions; risk factors, independent and dependent variables, and other kinds of variables; how to calculate and interpret measures of central tendency and variability; the normal curve; commonly used measures of association and what they mean; criteria that have been suggested for inferring causality from nonexperimental research; and different types of t-tests.

This book provides fundamental and practical knowledge about research methodology that is essential for health care chaplains, and students and professionals in other health care fields and the social sciences.

The chapters in this book were originally published as articles in the *Journal of Health Care Chaplaincy*.

Kevin J. Flannelly has over 150 peer-reviewed publications, including studies in various areas of psychology and articles about chaplaincy, clergy, research methods, and the association of religion with physical and mental health. He was the Editor-in-Chief of the *Journal of Health Care Chaplaincy* from 2008 through 2017.

Laura T. Flannelly has published articles on nursing, chaplaincy, and research methodology. She was an Associate Professor of Nursing at the University of Hawai'i at Mānoa, USA, where she taught psychiatric nursing in the graduate and undergraduate nursing programs.

Katherine R. B. Jankowski has co-authored articles in the *Journal of Health Care Chaplaincy*, the *Journal of Adult Development*, and the *Hispanic Journal of Behavioral Science*. Her research focuses on spirituality and adult development. She is an Adjunct Professor at Iona College, New Rochelle, USA.

Quantitative Research for Chaplains and Health Care Professionals

A Primer

Kevin J. Flannelly, Laura T. Flannelly and Katherine R. B. Jankowski

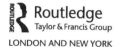
Routledge
Taylor & Francis Group

LONDON AND NEW YORK

First published 2019
by Routledge
2 Park Square, Milton Park, Abingdon, Oxon, OX14 4RN, UK

and by Routledge
52 Vanderbilt Avenue, New York, NY 10017, USA

First issued in paperback 2020

Routledge is an imprint of the Taylor & Francis Group, an informa business

© 2019 Taylor & Francis

British Library Cataloguing-in-Publication Data
A catalogue record for this book is available from the British Library

ISBN 13: 978-0-367-58325-5 (pbk)
ISBN 13: 978-1-138-35077-9 (hbk)

Typeset in ITC Garamond Std
by codeMantra

Publisher's Note
The publisher accepts responsibility for any inconsistencies that may have arisen during the conversion of this book from journal articles to book chapters, namely the possible inclusion of journal terminology.

Disclaimer
Every effort has been made to contact copyright holders for their permission to reprint material in this book. The publishers would be grateful to hear from any copyright holder who is not here acknowledged and will undertake to rectify any errors or omissions in future editions of this book.

Contents

CONTENTS

Citation Information

The chapters in this book were originally published in the *Journal of Health Care Chaplaincy*. When citing this material, please use the original page numbering for each article, as follows:

Chapter 1
Scientific Method and Its Application to Chaplaincy
Kevin J. Flannelly and Katherine R. B. Jankowski
Journal of Health Care Chaplaincy, volume 20, issue 1 (January 2014) pp. 1–2

Chapter 2
Research Designs and Making Causal Inferences from Health Care Studies
Kevin J. Flannelly and Katherine R. B. Jankowski
Journal of Health Care Chaplaincy, volume 20, issue 1 (January 2014) pp. 25–38

Chapter 3
Fundamentals of Measurement in Health Care Research
Laura T. Flannelly, Kevin J. Flannelly, and Katherine R. B. Jankowski
Journal of Health Care Chaplaincy, volume 20, issue 2 (April 2014) pp. 75–82

Chapter 4
Operational Definitions in Research on Religion and Health
Kevin J. Flannelly, Katherine R. B. Jankowski, and Laura T. Flannelly
Journal of Health Care Chaplaincy, volume 20, issue 2 (April 2014) pp. 83–91

Chapter 5
Independent, Dependent, and Other Variables in Healthcare and Chaplaincy Research
Laura T. Flannelly, Kevin J. Flannelly and Katherine R. B. Jankowski
Journal of Health Care Chaplaincy, volume 20, issue 4 (October 2014) pp. 161–170

Chapter 6
Measures of Central Tendency in Chaplaincy, Health Care, and Related Research
Katherine R. B. Jankowski and Kevin J. Flannelly
Journal of Health Care Chaplaincy, volume 21, issue 1 (January 2015)
pp. 39–49

Chapter 7
Measures of Variability in Chaplaincy, Health Care, and Related Research
Kevin J. Flannelly, Katherine R. B. Jankowski and Laura T. Flannelly
Journal of Health Care Chaplaincy, volume 21, issue 3 (July 2015)
pp. 122–130

Chapter 8
Studying Associations in Health Care Research
Kevin J. Flannelly, Laura T. Flannelly and Katherine R. B. Jankowski
Journal of Health Care Chaplaincy, volume 22, issue 3 (July 2016)
pp. 118–131

Chapter 9
The t-*test: An Influential Inferential Tool in Chaplaincy and Other Healthcare Research*
Katherine R. B. Jankowski, Kevin J. Flannelly and Laura T. Flannelly
Journal of Health Care Chaplaincy, volume 24, issue 1 (January 2018)
pp. 30–39

Chapter 10
Threats to the Internal Validity of Experimental and Quasi-Experimental Research in Healthcare
Kevin J. Flannelly, Laura T. Flannelly and Katherine R. B. Jankowski
Journal of Health Care Chaplaincy, volume 24, issue 3 (August 2018)
pp. 107–130

For any permission-related enquiries please visit:
http://www.tandfonline.com/page/help/permissions

Scientific Method and Its Application to Chaplaincy

KEVIN J. FLANNELLY and KATHERINE R. B. JANKOWSKI

The American philosopher Charles Sanders Peirce (1877) said there were four ways of knowing, or "fixing belief," as he called it (Kerlinger, 1973). The first is the method of tenacity in which people hold something to be true because they know it is true, and nothing can convince them that it is not true. The second is the method of authority, in which, as the name implies, people accept a proposition to be true because a powerful institution or other authority claims it is true. Peirce called the third way of knowing the *a priori* method because a proposition is accepted as being a self-evident truth. It also has been called the method of intuition, because one concludes a proposition is true on the basis of intuition; that is, it appears to be reasonable or logical. Peirce said some propositions are accepted without question or analysis *(a priori)* because they agree with reason, although they do not necessarily agree with experience (Kerlinger, 1973; Peirce, 1877).

The last method of "fixing belief" is the "method of science" or "scientific method." Scientific method, according to Peirce (1877), is predicated on the premise that: "There are real things, whose characters are entirely independent of our opinions about them…" (p. 10). Peirce did not think "fixing belief" using scientific method was reserved for scientists, and he thought that everyone should, and they often do, use scientific method in their everyday lives. Kerlinger (1973) similarly endorsed the general application of scientific method, saying it is "a special systematized form of all reflective thinking and inquiry" (p. 11).

Underwood (1957) said the purpose of scientific method was to describe and understand nature, and he thought the commonly made distinction between "pure" and "applied" science was a false dichotomy. Instead, he saw pure and applied science as ends of a continuum, in which the place of a research project along "this continuum is defined by the attitude of the research[er]" (Underwood, 1957, p. 9). A study that was recently published in the *Journal of Health Care Chaplaincy* (*JHCC*) illustrates the relative nature of this continuum (Gaudette & Jankowski, 2013). The study examined the association between spiritual beliefs and practices and general anxiety in a sample of palliative care patients. On the one hand, the study can be viewed as an example of applied research because the study's findings that spiritual beliefs and practices are associated with lower anxiety can be used to develop chaplain interventions to reduce patient anxiety. On the other hand, the study can be viewed as an example of pure (or basic) research because the findings contribute to our fundamental knowledge of the relationship between spirituality and mental health, which has theoretical as well as practical implications.

This issue of *JHCC* introduces the first article in the Journal's new section on Research Methodology. The section will feature an on-going series of articles about the application of scientific method in chaplaincy and related healthcare research. The first article describes different research designs and the degree to which one can draw causal inferences from their findings. However, research design is only one component of a research study that determines its quality, and the series will cover many other aspects of the research process. This series of articles on research aims to provide a quick reference for chaplains to prepare them to understand the research literature, to be active participants in research, and to identify and engage in evidence-based chaplaincy practices.

REFERENCES

Gaudette, H., & Jankowski, K. R. (2013). Spiritual coping and anxiety in palliative care patients: A pilot study. *Journal of Health Care Chaplaincy, 19*(4), 131–139.

Kerlinger, F. N. (1973). *Foundations of behavorial research* (2nd ed.). New York, NY: Holt, Rhinehart & Winston.

Peirce, C. S. (1877). The fixation of belief. *Popular Science Monthly, November*, 1–15.

Underwood, B. J. (1957). *Psychological research*. New York, NY: Appleton Century Crofts.

Research Designs and Making Causal Inferences from Health Care Studies

KEVIN J. FLANNELLY and KATHERINE R. B. JANKOWSKI

This article summarizes the major types of research designs used in healthcare research, including experimental, quasi-experimental, and observational studies. Observational studies are divided into survey studies (descriptive and correlational studies), case-studies and analytic studies, the last of which are commonly used in epidemiology: case-control, retrospective cohort, and prospective cohort studies. Similarities and differences among the research designs are described and the relative strength of evidence they provide is discussed. Emphasis is placed on five criteria for drawing causal inferences that are derived from the writings of the philosopher John Stuart Mill, especially his methods or canons. The application of the criteria to experimentation is explained. Particular attention is given to the degree to which different designs meet the five criteria for making causal inferences. Examples of specific studies that have used various designs in chaplaincy research are provided.

Traditionally, healthcare research has been divided into two categories: *observational* research and *experimental* research, or simply experimentation

TABLE 1 Research Designs in Descending Order of Their Strength of Evidence

---

Experimental Research (Experiments–Randomized Control Trials)
Quasi-Experimental Research
    Observational Research
    Analytic Studies
        Prospective Cohort
        Retrospective Cohort
        Case-Control
    Survey Studies
        Correlational (cross-sectional and longitudinal)
        Descriptive (cross-sectional)
    Case Studies

(Dawson-Saunders & Trapp, 1994; Mausner & Kramer, 1985). Observational research is a broad category that includes several different types of research designs, including surveys, case studies, and specific types of epidemiological study designs that will be discussed later (Dawson-Saunders & Trapp, 1994). A third type of research design is also recognized in health care and the social sciences (Cook & Campbell, 1979; Kleinbaum, Kupper, & Morgenstern, 1982; Macnee & McCabe, 2008), although it is ignored in many textbooks on health research: that is, quasi-experimental research (see Table 1).

OBSERVATIONAL RESEARCH

Observational research provides a fertile ground for thought. This type of research often yields evidence that supports questioning commonly accepted beliefs, and it can provide new insights and new ways of thinking about causes and effects. It is exceptionally helpful in the development of new theory and study of new fields of inquiry. Observational research has the potential to be done quickly, with uncomplicated designs, and minimal monetary investment.

    Survey studies collect information, or data, from individuals using questionnaires or face-to-face interviews. Interviews are typically used when it is important to delve more deeply into issues or individual experiences than can be done using standard questionnaires (Dawson-Saunders & Trapp, 1994). The purpose of the survey dictates the kinds of questions it asks. Social surveys usually collect information about people's attitudes and opinions about social issues, whereas health surveys collect information about height, weight, blood pressure, symptoms of disease, and so forth. Almost all survey studies collect information about the attributes or characteristics of the individuals that they survey, such as age, gender, and marital status. Naturally, these characteristics vary from person to person. A survey of U.S. adults, for example, may question people anywhere from 18 to 100 years of age. The same participants may be males or females, and they may be married, or unmarried. In scientific language, these attributes are called variables because the attributes vary along some dimension. Indeed, the scientific term for anything that varies along a dimension is a *variable*, including attitudes, opinions, and measures of health and health outcomes.

The first modern social survey study was conducted by interviewing household members in London during the 1880s. The survey's results appeared in the 1889 book, *Life and Labour of the People of London*, and a series of books that followed (Marsden & Wright, 2010). Social surveys have been ubiquitous in the United States since the 1950s, and U.S. health surveys have steadily increased since then, as well. Today, survey research is the most commonly used research method in the social sciences (except psychology), and it is widely used in the health sciences.

It is not surprising, therefore, that surveys are the most common type of study method used in chaplaincy research (Galek, Flannelly, Jankowski, & Handzo, 2011). During the last decade (2000–2009), survey studies in chaplaincy have explored a number of topics, asking: patients about their satisfaction with chaplaincy care; hospital administrators about the roles and functions of chaplains in their institutions; and chaplains about their interventions and the spiritual needs of their patients (Galek et al., 2011). Many survey studies related to chaplaincy fall into the category of *descriptive* studies, because they simply describe the attitudes, behaviors, health outcomes, and so forth of the people surveyed.

The *Journal of Health Care Chaplaincy* (*JHCC*) published a number of survey studies in the past few years that we think are good examples of *descriptive* studies. One is a survey that asked chaplains at several prominent U.S. hospitals about their access to medical records (Goldstein, Marin, & Umpierre, 2011). Another analyzed the survey responses of over 200 chaplains to questions about the challenges, rewards, and frustrations of working in the U.S. Veterans Health Administration (Beder & Yan, 2013). Large-scale descriptive studies have been used in epidemiology to measure the incidence and prevalence of diseases, other health problems, and behaviors in a population (Kleinbaum et al., 1982). Descriptive studies are mainly used in epidemiology when little is known about the occurrence or etiology (i.e., cause or origin) of a disease. Incidence and prevalence are different measures of the rate of occurrence or presence of diseases, among others, which will be discussed in a later article on research methodology.

The second major category of survey studies is the *correlational* study, which measures the correlations or relationships among different variables. Health researchers often look at the correlations between variables measuring personal characteristics and experiences and variables measuring health outcomes to see if the former are related to health outcomes. The first statistical procedure to measure correlations between variables was developed by Charles Darwin's cousin Francis Galton to measure inherited similarities in physical attributes (Galton, 1888). Galton's colleague, Karl Pearson developed the mathematical formula for the correlation coefficient, which is still used today (Dawson-Saunders & Trapp, 1994). The correlation coefficient measures the strength and direction of association between two variables.

When *descriptive* studies and *correlational* studies are conducted by surveying people at a certain point in time, they are called *cross-sectional* studies because their measures are recorded at a cross-section in time (Kleinbaum et al., 1982). As *cross-sectional* studies measure all of the study's variables at the same time they can only tell us how things are and what is occurring at the time the survey was conducted. Descriptive studies and correlational studies are often lumped together as cross-sectional studies in the medical literature, although correlational studies typically provide more information about relationships between variables.

JHCC has published several correlational studies in the past few years. A recent pilot study of spirituality and anxiety in palliative care patients is a particularly good example because it analyzed the collected data using a statistical procedure called correlation (Gaudette & Jankowski, 2013). Correlational analysis, which is the basis for the term correlational study, measures the degree that two things are related to, or associated with, each other. In this study, correlations were used to measure the degree to which: (a) anxiety was related to beliefs about God, and (b) anxiety was related to spiritual practices, such as meditation. The study also made limited use of a related statistical procedure developed by Galton and Pearson called regression analysis. An excellent example of the capacity of correlational studies to shed light on complex issues is a large-scale study of Swiss patients that used a regression analysis to examine the extent to which patient satisfaction with chaplaincy care was influenced by various factors, such as patient age, gender, religion, health status, and hospital length of stay (Winter-Pfandler & Morgenthaler, 2011). Correlation, regression, and other measures of association will be explained in later articles.

Analytic studies are a third category of *observational* studies that are employed in epidemiological research (Katz, 2001; Kleinbaum et al., 1982; Mausner & Kramer, 1985). The primary purposes of *analytic* studies are to identify risk factors associated with a disease and to estimate the degree to which these factors influence a disease. The term "risk factor" is used in epidemiology instead of "cause" to refer to a variable that is believed to contribute to the development of a disease (Kleinbaum et al.). The three major research designs of *analytic* studies are the *case-control* study, the *retrospective cohort* study, and the *prospective cohort* study (Katz; Kelsey, Thompson, & Evans, 1986; Kleinbaum et al.).

A *case-control* study assembles a group of people who have a disease, or other health outcome (the cases), and a group of similar people who do not have the disease (the controls), and compares the life histories of the individuals in the two groups to try to discover why the disease developed in the cases but not the controls (Dawson-Saunders & Trapp, 1994; Katz, 2001). The first *case-control* study in the United States appears to have been the investigation of an outbreak of scarlet fever in Flint Michigan in 1924. The cause of the outbreak was determined, surprisingly, to be ice cream (Morabia, 2013). Many case-control studies since then have attempted to trace the connection between chronic diseases and exposure to environmental risk factors that occurred years ago, which is a much more difficult task (Archer, 1988; Mezei & Kheifets, 2006; Teschke et al., 2002).

Cohort studies compare groups of people to determine what may have caused a disease or other health outcome. Whereas study participants in case-control studies are assigned to groups on the basis of a health outcome, such as lung cancer, participants in cohort studies are assigned to groups based on some factor that is suspected of being a precursor, or risk factor, for a health outcome. The cohort is simply a group of people with something in common who remain part of this studied group over time (Dawson-Saunders & Trapp, 1994). For instance, all the people who were born in a certain year, say 1995, would form the 1995 age-cohort. Commonly used cohorts in epidemiological studies are people working in particular industries or occupations (Kelsey et al., 1986). The purpose of cohort studies is to assess if past exposure (or lack of exposure) to health risks (e.g., cigarette smoking, or working with asbestos) predict some specified health outcomes—or other outcomes of interest (e.g., lung cancer) (Kelsey et al., 1986).

Like case-control studies, *retrospective cohort* studies look into the past to find the risks for disease, and study groups of people to look into the future to see if the outcome of interest occurs. While case-control studies and *retrospective cohort* studies try to determine how past situations and events affected current and future health outcomes, respectively, *prospective cohort* studies attempt to predict how current circumstances affect future outcomes. In *prospective cohort* studies, the intent is to identify groups before (or very soon after) one group is exposed to a health risk-factor. The groups are then followed into the future to see if the health outcome of interest emerges over time (Katz, 2001; Kelsey et al., 1986; Kleinbaum et al., 1982). The Framingham Heart Study, which began in 1948, was one of the first prospective studies conducted in the United States. This study, which coined the term "risk factor," examined blood pressure, cholesterol, smoking and other personal characteristics as risk factors for coronary heart disease in men (Berridge, Gorsky, & Mold, 2011; Kelsey et al.).

Case studies, which have a long history in medicine, form the fourth and last major category of observational research. *Case studies* also have a long history in chaplaincy. Anton Boisen used them as teaching tools in clinical pastoral education (as cited in Asquith, 1980). A case study is generally defined as an in-depth investigation of one person, institution, or social group (Merriam, 1988; Rubinson & Neutens, 1987). Case studies of patients are still used in medicine, and they can be an important first step in developing more methodologically sophisticated studies (Dawson-Saunders & Trapp, 1994; Fitchett, 2011; Kelsey et al., 1986).

Fitchett (2011) has argued that they are an ideal form of research for chaplains. In the past three years, JHCC has published three case studies of patients, which readers should find useful. The first is the case of a woman with advanced metastatic breast cancer (Cooper, 2011), the second is the case of woman with recurrent leukemia (King, 2012), and the third is the case of a male out-patient with Parkinson's disease who was being treated for depression (Risk, 2013).

EXPERIMENTAL RESEARCH

Experimental research is often considered to be the more complicated type of research even though this is not always true (Cook & Campbell, 1979). Direct manipulation of environmental factors often occurs in experimental research, and the interference with, and manipulation of, environmental factors requires careful thought about ethics, especially when human beings are involved as participants in the research. *Experimental* research can provide the best support for cause and effect explanatory relationships (Campbell & Stanley, 1963; Greenhalgh, 2001).

Experimental research in medicine was formalized in the mid nineteenth century through the work of Claude Bernard (Bernard, 1865/1957), although medical research had been conducted for centuries prior to that (Singer, 1950). A few years before Bernard's book was published, the philosopher John Stuart Mill (1859) published his ideas about scientific reasoning, experimental methods, and inferring causality from research. For our purposes, Mill's key proposals may be summarized as five criteria for drawing causal inferences from experimentation (Mill, himself, did not number them.). First, the presumptive cause, or causal agent, must precede the effect in time. The cause must occur before the effect. Second, the effect must occur whenever the presumptive cause is present (Mills' Method of Agreement). The effect always happens if the cause has occurred. Third, the effect must not occur when the presumptive cause is absent (Mills' Method of Difference). Fourth, the presumptive cause must be isolated from other potential causes of the effect. Fifth, to ensure that the presumptive cause is isolated from all other potential causes, it must be produced artificially, which in this situation precludes observing the natural occurrence of the causal agent.

Mill (1859) proposed two other methods for identifying causal relationships:[1] The Method of Concomitant Variations and the Methods of Residues. Mill also recognized that there may be multiple causes of an effect. Current statistical methods can help identify multiple causes, but we are not going to treat this topic here.

The renowned scientist Louis Pasteur was conducting studies that employed Mill's experimental methods around the same time that Mill was writing about them (Singer, 1950). A famous experiment by Pasteur was designed to test the theory of spontaneous generation of gas. It can be viewed as a simple test of whether fermentation requires bacteria to occur. To test this, Pasteur created a solution, in which bacteria normally produced fermentation, in a sealed flask. Next, he heated the flask to kill any bacteria and other living matter already in the flask. Then, he waited for months to see if fermentation occurred when no bacteria were present (the method of difference). The method of difference confirmed that fermentation (the effect) did not occur without the presence of live bacteria (the causal agent). When Pasteur eventually unsealed the flask to expose it to bacteria (the causal agent) in the air, fermentation (the effect) occurred in the flask within hours (the method of agreement).[2] Mill strongly advised that researchers use both methods, in what he called the Joint Method of Agreement and Difference, and this is what Pasteur did sequentially.

Modern experimental research adheres to Mill's five criteria to make it possible to draw causal inferences from experimental results (Plutchik, 1968). The first criterion is applied in experimentation by presenting or administering an experimental treatment (Mill's presumptive cause), and then measuring its effect or outcome. Thus, the presumptive cause precedes the intended effect. In human research, the outcome of interest is usually measured before the treatment is administered, to see if it is already present to some degree (Campbell, 1957; Campbell & Stanley, 1963).

The second and third criteria are applied by using Mill's Joint Method of Agreement and Difference, simultaneously, in which some participants receive the treatment (the experimental condition) and some participants to do not receive the treatment (the control condition) (Campbell, 1957; Campbell & Stanley, 1963). The fourth criterion is followed by carefully trying to control for variations in environmental variables that may affect the outcome (called extraneous variables) other than the experimental treatment (Campbell, 1957; Kidder & Judd, 1959). Human and animal experimentation further controls for extraneous variables, in the form of personal differences, by randomly assigning participants to the experimental and control conditions (Edwards, 1985; Kidder & Judd).

The fifth criterion is an inherent part of experimentation in that the presence or absence of a treatment (which is somewhat oddly referred to as the independent variable) is artificially manipulated by the researcher, as is the case when the treatment is a surgical procedure (Kleinbaum et al., 1982). The level of treatment is also manipulated in many experiments, such as drug treatments that consists of different doses of a drug (Kleinbaum et al.), In such experiments, one might predict that the strength of the outcome would vary by dose, which is an example of Mill's Method of Concomitant Variations (Mill, 1859).

Adherence to these five criteria is what defines an experiment (Plutchik, 1968). In modern language, the defining characteristics of experiments are said to be: manipulation of the independent variable (treatment), randomization of participants to conditions, and control of extraneous variables (Kidder & Judd, 1959). Experiments in medicine that adhere to these principles have come to be called "randomized control trials" (RCTs) (Dawson-Saunders & Trapp, 1994; Katz, 2001).

A study by Bay and his colleagues (Bay, Beckman, Trippi, Gunderman, & Terry, 2008) is one of a few published experimental studies in the chaplaincy research literature. Positive health outcomes, such as positive religious coping and reduced negative religious coping were studied in cardiac patients over a short period of time. Many controls were instituted to isolate the effects of a chaplaincy intervention on cardiac patients. The chaplain's intervention followed an exact schedule and one chaplain delivered the intervention. The participants' characteristics were controlled, including the requirements that participants speak and understand English, that participants have only one of two kinds of heart surgery, and that participants agree to be randomly assigned to the treatment condition (chaplaincy) or control condition (no chaplaincy). Participants were required to attend all the chaplain's meetings and complete all the questionnaires. Increased positive religious coping and reduced negative religious coping were found in the treatment group compared to the control group. A more detailed discussion will be found on the possible conclusions drawn from these findings in a future article delving deeper into experimental design.

QUASI-EXPERIMENTAL RESEARCH

The term quasi-experimental was introduced in 1963 in the context of conducting research in educational and social settings (Campbell & Stanley, 1963). Campbell and Stanley's book explored the problems that limit one's ability to make causal inferences from "true" experimental studies and studies that lack some of the key features of "true" experiments, a topic that was initially addressed by Campbell (1957). Although some people refer to quasi-experiments as natural experiments, quasi-experimental designs are used to study the effects of many things that are not acts of nature. The term quasi-experiment or quasi-experimental design is typically used to describe studies in which the independent variable is not manipulated by the researcher and the "participants" are not randomly assigned to conditions (Kleinbaum et al., 1982). However, it also applies to research in which there is no control group, such as quality improvement research.

Although there is little available information on the extent to which quasi-experiments are used in medicine or other healthcare fields, a 2005 review of research on infectious diseases identified 73 quasi-experimental studies that were published in three journals in just two years (Harris,

Lautenbach, & Perencevich, 2005). Over three-quarters of the studies did not have a control group.

A study of students in clinical pastoral education (CPE) published in *JHCC* is a good example of a quasi-experiment (Jankowski, Vanderwerker, Murphy, Montonye, & Ross, 2008). Student growth in chaplaincy skills was assessed for groups of students taking a shorter intensive unit or a longer, extended unit of CPE. Students completed questionnaires at the beginning and the end of each unit of CPE, which measured their pastoral skills, emotional intelligence, and self-reflection. Controlling for major demographic variables, and the two types of CPE units, students with no prior CPE and fewer years of professional ministry, were found to experience more positive change in their pastoral skills. Controlling for demographic variables, students in intensive CPE experienced greater increases in emotional intelligence and self-reflection. However, the ability to draw causal conclusions from the study is limited by the lack of a control group and the fact that students were not randomly assigned to the two types of CPE units. While differences in the demographic characteristics of the two groups were controlled for statistically, other, unmeasured characteristics of students in the intensive units could account for the findings.

MAKING CAUSAL INFERENCES FROM RESEARCH

The types of research we have discussed, traditionally, have been viewed as a hierarchy with respect to the quality of evidence they provide for assessing causal inferences (Greenhalgh, 2001). Experimentation forms the top of the hierarchy because it establishes the temporal order needed to infer causation, and controls for other alternative explanations of what might have caused the observed outcome. The goal of experimentation is to reduce, if not eliminate, the possibility of some alternative explanation for the apparent effect of treatment, other than the treatment (Edwards, 1985; Katz, 2001).

If the expected outcome is observed in the experimental group and not the control group one can logically conclude that the outcome is due to the experimental treatment. The possibility that the outcome is attributable to other variables that could have affected the participants at the same time as the treatment was administered is eliminated to the degree that the experimental and control conditions are identical except for the treatment (Edwards, 1985; Kidder & Judd, 1959). Because participants are randomly assigned to conditions, or groups, the differences in outcomes between the groups cannot be due to differences in the personal characteristics of the participants in the groups because random assignment should ensure that the characteristics of the participants are, on average, comparable in the groups (Edwards, 1985; Greenhalgh, 2001; Mausner & Kramer, 1985). Although Mill thought multiple experiments, or experimental trials, in which a presumptive cause was present or absent, might be required to be able to determine causality, experiments in modern medicine and other fields often consist of a single trial during which the participants in the experimental condition receive the experimental treatment (Greenhalgh, 2001).

Quasi-experiments are lower on the hierarchy for several reasons. To the degree the temporal order of the presumptive cause and the observed outcome can be established, the temporal order required for inferring causality is not a problem. However, the nature of quasi-experiments poses several threats to the ability to infer cause-effects relationships from them. Because the researcher does not manipulate the independent variable (or treatment), the observed outcome could be the result of something that occurred about the same time as the presumptive cause. This possibility is not easily dismissed because quasi-experiments, unlike experiments, do not control for extraneous variables. The lack of random assignment of participants to experimental and control poses another threat since, without random assignment, the differential outcomes could be due to differences between participants in the conditions. Some quasi-experiments lack any group with which the experimental effects can be compared.

Cross-sectional surveys and case-studies are traditionally placed at the bottom of the hierarchy. The problem with cross-sectional surveys is that they cannot determine the temporal order of events that is needed to infer a cause-effect relationship between two variables, because the personal characteristics of survey participants and their health outcomes are measured at the same point in time (Kelsey et al., 1986; Mausner & Kramer, 1985). This inability of survey studies to establish the temporal relationship required to draw causal inferences can be corrected by conducting surveys of the same individuals at two or more points in time. This type of survey research is called a longitudinal study rather than a cross-sectional study.

Case-studies are placed at the low end of the hierarchy for two reasons: their inability to draw causal inferences and their lack of generalizability. First, case-studies of patients are very rarely, if ever, conducted before the patient has a disease or other health problem, so case-studies do not provide a time-line by which to determine whether a cause-effect relationship exists. Second, it is often difficult to generalize the circumstances of a particular person to other people. However, case-studies may be used to study the effects of treatment, regardless of the disease etiology, a point that is often lost in the medical literature. Moreover, as previously mentioned, case studies can be helpful in the development of more sophisticated studies of a topic (Dawson-Saunders & Trapp, 1994; Fitchett, 2011; Kelsey et al., 1986).

Analytical studies fall toward the middle of hierarchy. The case-control study is ranked just above cross-sectional surveys and case studies in the hierarchy because their design permits them to differentiate between cause and effect by demonstrating that exposure to some risk factor occurred prior to a disease. However, as the study may be conducted years after the exposure, documenting the temporal relationship between risk factors and health outcomes may be problematic (Kelsey et al., 1986; Mausner & Kramer, 1985). The required documentation of exposure to the risk factor, and/or the onset of the disease may be inadequate because of poor recoding keeping or poor memories of the events (Kelsey et al., 1986; Mausner & Kramer).

Even when the temporal relationship can be properly established, the causal link between exposure and disease is not conclusive. Case-control studies assume that the cases and controls are members of the same population, who only differ from each other with respect to exposure to the risk factor. If this is not true, the putative risk factor may not be the cause of the outcome, since the outcome could be the result of something else that is similar to the cases but different between the cases and controls (Kleinbaum et al., 1982). This was the basic criticism of the case-control studies that identified cigarette smoking as a risk factor for lung cancer. The alternative explanation was that people who smoke and people who develop lung cancer share some common characteristic, other than smoking, that was the cause of the lung cancer (Dawson-Saunders & Trapp, 1994). Despite their weaknesses, case-control studies are useful for studying rare diseases and identifying possible risk factors (Kelsey et al., 1986).

Retrospective cohort-studies, many of which have examined health problems associated with workplace risk factors (Kelsey et al., 1986), form the next rung of the hierarchy (Greenhalgh, 2001). Generally, cohort studies provide stronger evidence for cause and effect between risks and outcomes than case-control studies because the selection of cases is done before the adverse health outcome is observed (Dawson-Saunders & Trapp, 1994; Kelsey et al.). Hence, at least in theory, they can establish the temporal order required to draw causal inferences. However, because they attempt to look back in time to establish the temporal relationship needed to determine the cause-effect relationship between a risk factors and disease, they face some of the same problems as case-control studies. For example, they may not be able to (a) document the temporal relationship between risk factors and outcomes, or (b) identify and measure variables that may be risk factors for the disease apart from the supposed risk factor. Finally, the selection of the appropriate controls can be difficult, since the controls should be representative of the general population overall, and with respective to exposure to the risk factor (Kelsey et al., 1986; Mausner & Kramer, 1985).

Prospective cohort studies are ranked above retrospective cohort-studies for a number of reasons, based on the fact that they are truly longitudinal, and observe individuals across time rather than trying to recreate their life histories (Mausner & Kramer, 1985). The first reason, and the major advantage of prospective studies, is that the timing of exposure to risk factors and disease onset can be clearly established for individuals in the study (Mausner & Kramer). Second, they also are less likely to miss shared variables among the cases other than the risk factor that might cause the outcome, although the possibility of alternative causal agents always exist in observational studies (Dawson-Saunders & Trapp, 1994). Once such shared variables are identified, their effects can be controlled statistically; therefore, the effects of the hypothesized risk factor can be isolated from their effects on the health outcome. Third, prospective cohort studies can assess multiple health outcomes because they start at the time of exposure to the risk factor and follow individuals into the future, during which time more than one effect of the exposure may emerge (Kelsey et al., 1986; Mausner & Kramer, 1985).

CONCLUSIONS

Healthcare research efforts begin humbly, through diligent observations of healthcare provision, utilization, and/or outcomes. These observations become increasingly more complex if the researcher intends to identify cause and effect relationships, whether to reduce or prevent disease or to improve education and practice. Attention must be paid to many variables, such as participants' characteristics, the setting of the research, and the timing of events. Time is crucial to establish cause and effect, and research findings should always be evaluated with attention to the criteria for drawing causal inferences from experimentation and other types of research. Knowledge of research methods and reasoning will decrease the likelihood that researchers will fall into the error of making cause and effect statements that are not justified by the methodology employed in a study.

NOTES

1. Collectively, Mill's five methods have been called Mill's Canons (Katz, 2001).
2. The fact that fermentation did not occur until air-borne bacteria entered the flask was taken as evidence that spontaneous generation had not occurred, which so undermined the theory of spontaneous generation that is was no longer taken seriously in scientific circles.

REFERENCES

Archer, V. E. (1988). Lung cancer risks of underground miners: cohort and case-control studies. *Yale Journal of Biology and Medicine, 61*(3), 183–193.

Asquith, G. R. (1980). The case study method of Anton T. Boisen. *Journal of Pastoral Care, 34*(2), 84–94.

Bay, P. S., Beckman, D., Trippi, J., Gunderman, R., & Terry, C. (2008). The effect of pastoral care services on anxiety, depression, hope, religious coping, and religious problem solving styles: A randomized controlled study. *Journal of Religion and Health, 47*(1), 57–69.

Beder, J., & Yan, G. W. (2013). VHA Chaplains: challenges, roles, rewards, and frustrations of the work. *Journal of Health Care Chaplaincy, 19*(2), 54–65.

Bernard, C. (1865/1957). *An introduction to the study of experimental medicine.* New York, NY: Dover Publications.

Berridge, V., Gorsky, M., & Mold, A. (2011). *Public health in history.* Berkshire, UK: Open University Press.

Campbell, D. T. (1957). Factors relevant to the validity of experiments in social settings *Psychological Review, 54*(4), 297–312.

Campbell, D. T., & Stanley, J. C. (1963). *Experimental and quasi-experimental designs for research.* Chicago, IL: Rand McNally

Cook, T. D., & Campbell, D. T. (1979). *Quasi-experimentation: Design & analysis issues for field settings.* Boston, MA: Houghton Mifflin.

Cooper, R. S. (2011). Case study of a chaplain's spiritual care for a patient with advanced metastatic breast cancer. *Journal of Health Care Chaplaincy, 17*(1–2), 19–37.

Dawson-Saunders, B., & Trapp, R. G. (1994). *Basic and clinical biostatistics* (2nd ed.). Norwalk, CT: Appleton & Lange.

Edwards, A. L. (1985). *Experimental design in psychological research* (Fifth Ed.). New York, NY: Harper & Rowe.

Fitchett, G. (2011). Making our case(s). *Journal of Health Care Chaplaincy, 17*(1–2), 3–18.

Galek, K., Flannelly, K. J., Jankowski, K. R., & Handzo, G. F. (2011). A methodological analysis of chaplaincy research: 2000–2009. *Journal of Health Care Chaplaincy, 17*(3–4), 126–145.

Galton, F. (1888). Co-relations and their measurement, chiefly from anthropometrics data. *Proceedings of the Royal Society of London, 45*, 135–145.

Gaudette, H., & Jankowski, K. R. (2013). Spiritual coping and anxiety in palliative care patients: A pilot study. *Journal of Health Care Chaplaincy, 19*(4), 131–139.

Goldstein, H. R., Marin, D., & Umpierre, M. (2011). Chaplains and access to medical records. *Journal of Health Care Chaplaincy, 17*(3–4), 162–168.

Greenhalgh, T. (2001). *How to read a paper: The basics of evidence based medicine.* London: BMJ Books.

Harris, A. D., Lautenbach, E., & Perencevich, E. (2005). A systematic review of quasi-experimental study designs in the fields of infection control and antibiotic resistance. *Clinical Infectious Disiseases, 41*(1), 77–82.

Jankowski, K. R. B., Vanderwerker, L. C., Murphy, K. M., Montonye, M., & Ross, A. M. (2008). Change in pastoral skills, emotional intelligence, self-reflection, and social desirability across a unit of CPE. *Journal of Health Care Chaplaincy, 15*(2), 132–148.

Katz, D. L. (2001). *Clinical epidemiology & evidence-based medicine.* Thousand Oaks, CA: Sage Publications.

Kelsey, J., Thompson, W. D., & Evans, A. S. (1986). *Methods in observational epidemiology.* New York, NY: Oxford University Press.

Kidder, L. H., & Judd, C. M. (1959). *Research methods in social relations* (Fifth Ed.). Fort Worth, TX: Holt, Rinehart & Winston.

King, S. D. (2012). Facing fears and counting blessings: A case study of a chaplain's faithful companioning a cancer patient. *Journal of Health Care Chaplaincy, 18*(1–2), 3–22.

Kleinbaum, D. G., Kupper, L. L., & Morgenstern, H. (1982). *Epidemiolic research: Principles and quantitative methods.* New York, NY: Van Nostrand Reinhold.

Macnee, C. L., & McCabe, S. (2008). *Understanding nursing research* (2nd ed.). Philadephia, PA: Lippincott, Williams & Wilkins.

Marsden, P. V., & Wright, J. D. (2010). Survey research and social science: History, current practice, and future prospects. In P. V. Marsden & J. D. Wright (Eds.), *Handbook of survey research* (2nd ed., pp. 3–25). Bingley, UK: Emerald Group Publishing.

Mausner, J., & Kramer, S. (1985). *Epidemiology: An introductory text* (2nd ed.). Philadelphia, PA: W.P. Saunders.

Merriam, A. B. (1988). *Case study research in eduation: A qualitative approach*. San Franciso, CA: Jossey-Bass.

Mezei, G., & Kheifets, L. (2006). Selection bias and its implications for case-control studies: a case study of magnetic field exposure and childhood leukaemia. *International Journal of Epidemiology, 35*(2), 397–406.

Mill, J. S. (1859). *A system of logic, ratiocinative and inductive; bring a connected view of the principles of evidence and the methods of scientific investigation*. New York: Harper & Brothers.

Morabia, A. (2013). Snippets from the past: Is Flint, Michigan, the birthplace of the case-control study? *American Journal of Epidemiology, [Epub ahead of print]*.

Plutchik, R. (1968). *Foundations of experimental research*. New York, NY: Harper & Rowe.

Risk, J. L. (2013). Building a new life: A chaplain's theory based case study of chronic illness. *Journal of Health Care Chaplaincy, 19*(3), 81–98.

Rubinson, L., & Neutens, J. J. (1987). *Research techniques in the health sciences*. New York, NY: Macmillan.

Singer, C. (1950). *A history of biology* (Reviseded.). New York, NY: Henry Schuman.

Teschke, K., Olshan, A. F., Daniels, J. L., De Roos, A. J., Parks, C. G., Schulz, M., ... Vaughn, T. L. (2002). Occupational exposure assessment in case-control studies: Opportunities for improvement. *Occupational and Environmental Medicine, 59*(9), 575–934.

Winter-Pfandler, U., & Morgenthaler, C. (2011). Patients' satisfaction with health care chaplaincy and affecting factors: An exploratory study in the German part of Switzerland. *Journal of Health Care Chaplaincy, 17*(3–4), 146–161.

Fundamentals of Measurement in Health Care Research

LAURA T. FLANNELLY, KEVIN J. FLANNELLY, and
KATHERINE R. B. JANKOWSKI

This article discusses levels of measurement and their application to research and practice in health care. The concept of levels of measurement was codified in a seminal article by S. S. Stevens in 1946 that defined four levels of measurement: nominal scales, which label and classify cases (objects and individuals) and assign them to categories; ordinal scales, which rank cases on some attribute; interval scales, which have equal intervals for measuring attributes; and ratio scales, which have equal intervals and a natural zero point. The rules that apply to each level of measurement are presented and the mathematical operations that can be performed on them are explained. The similarities and differences among the four types of scales are discussed and examples of their use in health care and other contexts are described.

"It's a man!" exclaimed Dorothy in the *Wizard of Oz,* when she first recognized the tin man as more than a statue. This memorable line from a memorable movie is a great example of how something as basic as naming can change everything. This section of our series on research will detail the importance of specificity in our measurement as it pertains to health care phenomena.

Two related issues about the measurement and meaning of scientific concepts were raised in the 1930s and 1940s, which are still relevant today. One issue arose in the field of physics (Bridgman, 1927, 1938, 1945), and the other arose from the psychological field of psychophysics (Stevens, 1946). The first issue, which is the topic of the companion article about operational definitions, addresses how scientific concepts are defined. The second issue, which addresses how scientific concepts are quantified (the measurement of concepts), is the topic of this article.

Stevens' 1946 article about the measurement of scientific concepts is the seminal paper on the topic: "On the Theory of Scales of Measurement" (Stevens, 1946). Stevens was an early advocate of the application of operational definitions in psychophysics—the psychological perception of physical sensations (Stevens, 1975)—and psychology, at large (Stevens, 1935). His thinking on this issue, no doubt, influenced his thinking about the measurement of concepts, since he thought both definition and measurement entailed the specification of empirical operations (Stevens, 1935, 1946). In the broadest sense, Stevens considered measurement to be the assignment of numbers to objects or events according a set of rules.

Stevens (1946) defined four levels of measurement (nominal, ordinal, interval and ratio levels), and his article explains the rules that govern them. The four levels of measurement form a hierarchy in which each higher level encompasses the characteristics of the preceding level, in addition to having some additional properties of its own (Bailey, 1987; Kerlinger, 1973; Polit & Hungler, 1989). Notably, there also is a hierarchy with respect to the mathematical operations that can be performed on data reflecting each level of measurement (Bailey, 1987; Kerlinger; Polit & Hungler).

NOMINAL SCALES

The nominal scale is the lowest level of measurement, in which names or labels are assigned to objects (cases). These names classify object characteristics, and objects can then be put into categories. We use nominal scales in everyday life when we identify people as males, females, Catholics, Protestants, nurses, chaplains, and so on. The demographic characteristics of research participants are often reported on a nominal scale, for example, blood type, gender, occupation, and religious denomination. Nominal scales are the simplest form of measurement because they simply classify cases (i.e., people and objects) into categories (Bailey, 1987; Kerlinger, 1973).

The requirements for nominal measurement are that the categories must be distinct, mutually exclusive, and exhaustive (Bailey, 1987; Rubinson & Neutens, 1987). By exhaustive, we mean that there is an appropriate category for each case. By mutually exclusive, we mean that each case appropriately fits only one category. Each case has a category (exhaustive) but only one category (mutual exclusiveness) into which it fits. For example, a person's blood type, O positive, puts them into only one category and no other blood type category applies.

Beyond assigning cases to membership in a category (A−, B+, O+), nominal measurement provides no additional information about the attributes of a variable. Using another example, assigning people into categories by their occupation (e.g., store clerk, nurse, or teacher) tells us nothing about how good they are at their job. Since nominal measurement involves naming and categorizing, the categories themselves and the cases in them have no numerical value. However, we can count the number of cases in each category, and we can see if there are more cases in one category or another. Additionally, if we look at two different categories at the same time, such as gender and occupation, we can gather more meaningful information. If we wanted to know if there are more female nurses than male nurses at a hospital, or more female doctors than male doctors, we would simultaneously look at the gender and occupations of the hospital staff to find the answer.

Apart from counting cases, no mathematical operations can be performed on nominal data, although the counts (or frequencies as they are called) can be used to calculate proportions, such as percentages. A study by Beder and Yan (2013) in the *Journal of Health Care Chaplaincy* illustrates the reporting of the common nominal variables in a research article. Table 1 of the study shows the number and percentage of chaplains employed by the Veterans Health Administration who responded to a survey, by their gender, race, religion, and employment status. A study by Vanderwerker, Flannelly, et al. (2008) is of particular interest because it employed nominal scales related to referrals to chaplains. One categorized the sources of referrals to chaplains (e.g., nurses, doctors, a patient's relatives) and the other categorized the reasons for referrals (e.g., anxiety, grief, or spiritual distress). Then, the study simultaneously looked at the sources and reasons for referrals to see whether hospital staff and family members referred patients to chaplains for different reasons.

In addition to demographic data, nominal measurement is common in medical research and practice since patients and other individuals are often considered to be cases based on the presence or absence of a disease diagnosis, a risk factor, or a treatment outcome (Dawson-Saunders & Trappan, 1994). A common use of nominal measurement in medicine is the case versus no case classification, in which a "case" is coded 1 and "no case" is coded as 0. One could just as reasonably code them 1 and 2 because they do not imply actual numerical values. However, coding them as 1 and 0 is intuitive, and makes it easy to count the number or cases, and hence, to calculate the proportion of cases, which is a very useful measure in medicine and epidemiology.

ORDINAL SCALES

Ordinal scales are similar to nominal scales in that they consist of mutually exclusive and exhaustive categories but, unlike nominal scales, each category of the scale expresses a different value. Ordinal scales rank objects and people (cases) in terms of their relative value on some attribute. The rank places the cases in an order to indicate they are "more than" or "less than" one another on the attribute, such as oldest, next oldest, and youngest (Ellis, 1998; Kerlinger, 1973). The key feature of ordinal measurement is that the ranks follow a specific order, but there is no assumption about the distances between each rank. For example, you might rank your five favorite movies on a scale of 1 to 5, with 1 being the one you like the most, 2 being the one you like second most, 3 being the one you like third most, etc. But, this ranking does not indicate how much more you like one movie compared to any other. It would make no difference if you ranked them the opposite way, with 5 being your favorite movie and 1 being your least favorite movie.

A familiar example of ordinal measurement is the ranking of military officers, which are, from the highest to lowest rank: general, colonel, major, captain, and lieutenant. However, one cannot quantify the distance one rank is from another, although higher ranking officers clearly have more power and authority. There are, of course, finer distinctions among military ranks than those listed here (Besterman-Dahan et al., 2012)

A more familiar example of an ordinal scale for most people is the academic ranking of a graduating class. The valedictorian is the person ranked first in the graduating class and the salutatorian is ranked second in the class, based on their grade point average (GPA). If the class consists of 50 students, each of the other students would be ranked from 3rd to 50th, based on their GPA. However, there is no reason to assume that the difference in GPA between the 1st and 2nd ranked students is the same as the difference in GPA between the 3rd and 4th ranked students, or that the difference is the same between the 49th and 50th ranked students. Ordinal numbers indicate rank order and nothing more (Ellis, 1998; Kerlinger, 1973). Rankings do not indicate absolute quantities, nor do they indicate that the intervals between the ranks are equal on whatever attribute is being measured, such as academic performance.

Polit and Hungler (1989) provide an excellent example of the use of an ordinal scale in health care, in which a patient's ability to perform activities of daily living was scored from 1 to 4: 1 = completely dependent; 2 = needs another person's assistance; 3 = needs mechanical assistance; and 4 = completely independent. All persons assigned a score of 4, then, are equivalent in their ability to function to others with the same score, and they have higher functioning than individuals assigned a score of 3. All persons with a score of 2 have lower functioning than persons with a score of 3 and higher functioning than persons with a score of 1.

Ordinal scales are commonly used in medicine to indicate the severity of a disease and/or the type of therapy that is appropriate (Dawson-Saunders & Trappan, 1994). Tumors, for example are staged according to their degree of development, in which a higher stage is worse than a lower stage with respect to prognosis. Like the stages of cancer, the progression of kidney and other diseases are labeled with higher stages designating more advanced disease progression.

INTERVAL SCALES

Interval scales have all of the characteristics of nominal and ordinal scales, and more. Interval scales are sometimes called equal interval scales because equal intervals are what make interval measurement different from ordinal measurement. Unlike ordinal scales, the numerical values of interval scales represent equal distances between the units of measurement (Bailey, 1987; Ellis, 1998; Kerlinger, 1973). Whereas ordinal scales only indicate that a person ranks higher or lower than another person on some attribute, interval scales indicate how much higher or lower one person is from another person on a variable in units of equal magnitude. SAT scores provide a common example. Obviously, a score of 600 is higher than a score of 550, and a score of 550 is higher than 500. More importantly, however, the difference between 600 and 550 (50 points) is equivalent to the difference between 550 and 500 (50 points) on an interval scale (Polit & Hungler, 1989).

Whatever the amount of difference between two scores is, this difference is always the same wherever it falls on an interval scale (Bailey, 1987). This characteristic is true of both the Fahrenheit and Celsius (or centigrade) temperature scales. Although the Fahrenheit and Celsius scales have different units of measurement, within each scale a difference of 10° (degrees) means the same thing no matter where it is located in the scale. The 10° difference in temperature between 70° and 60° represents the same difference in magnitude as the 10° difference in temperature between 40° and 30°, or between 20° and 10°.

Because the units of measurement are equal on an interval scale, addition and subtraction can be performed on the units of the scale. Although it makes no sense to add or subtract ranks, such as the rankings of a graduating class, one can add or subtract actual grade point averages (GPAs). Thus, one can meaningfully interpret the difference in the GPA (or the SAT scores) of the valedictorian and the salutatorian, or between any of the other students in the class. In doing so, we would expect the difference in GPA between the valedictorian and the salutatorian to be quite small $(4.0 - 3.9 = 0.1)$, and the difference in GPA between the 98th and 99th ranked students also to be quite small $(1.1 - 1.0 = .1)$. In this instance, the equal difference in values at the high and low ends of the scales mean the same thing, just as they do for SAT scores.

The ability to add and subtract scores on an interval scale is what makes this scale attractive to educators and psychologists, and interval scales which measure attitudes, tend to be very common in the social sciences and the behavioral health sciences (Rubinson & Neutens, 1987). Whether one is measuring academic achievement or self-ratings of health, the additivity of interval scales allows educators and researchers to calculate total scores from their measurements. This property of interval scales makes them much more useful and informative than ordinal scales. However, there is a major short-coming of interval scales; they lack a true zero point. There is no real complete absence of any graded effort for a GPA, or the complete absence of temperature as measured on the Fahrenheit and Celsius scales. Thus, one cannot say that a GPA of 3.8 is twice as high as GPA of 1.9, or a SAT score of 600 is three times greater than a SAT score of 200. One cannot say that a temperature of 80° on either of the thermometers is 2 times higher than 40°, 4 times higher than 20°, or 8 times higher than 10° (Kerlinger, 1973; Rubinson & Neutens, 1987).

RATIO SCALES

The highest level of measurement is ratio measurement (Bailey, 1987; Kerlinger, 1973; Polit & Hungler, 1989). In addition to having the characteristics of nominal, ordinal, and interval scales, ratio scales have an absolute, true zero that has an empirical meaning. The values of a ratio scale represent equal units of magnitude on a variable, and the zero point of a ratio scale represents the point at which the variable literally does not exist. All measures of length, volume, and time can be measured on ratio scales (Bailey; Kerlinger, 1973; Polit & Hungler). Duration of chaplains' visits is, for instance, a ratio measurement (Vanderwerker, Handzo, Fogg, & Overvold, 2008).

Height, weight, and age are common examples of ratio scales. Age, for example, clearly has the characteristics of an interval scale since one year is equivalent to one year at any age. Therefore, differences in age are equivalent at any age. Obviously, there is a 3-year difference between a 59-year-old person and a 56-year-old, and a 3-year difference between a 17-year-old and 14-year-old (although the mother of a 14-year-old might beg to differ). Like any measure of time, age also has a real, or absolute zero point (Bailey, 1987); we cannot be any younger than zero.

Since ratio scales have an absolute or natural zero, all arithmetic operations can be performed on them (Bailey, 1987; Kerlinger, 1973; Polit & Hungler, 1989). This includes multiplication and division, which cannot be performed on the other measurement scales. Ratio scale numbers can be expressed as ratio relationships, as the name ratio scale implies (Kerlinger, 1973). In the case of the variable age, for example, this means that age 80 is 2 times older than age 40, and 4 times older than age 20. Although the Fahrenheit and Celsius temperature scales do not have a natural zero point, the Kelvin scale does, so temperatures on the Kelvin scale can be expressed as ratios. Zero degrees Kelvin (0° K) is the equivalent of − 273°C and −460° F. On the Fahrenheit scale, water freezes at 32° F and boils at 212° F, so it would appear that the boiling point of water is 6.625 times higher than the freezing point of water. However, since the zero point on the Fahrenheit scale is artificial, this comparison is not only misleading, it is mistaken. In reality, the boiling point of water is only 1.366 times higher than the freezing point of water, which are 373° K and 273° K, respectively, on the Kelvin scale.

Most variables that measure length, volume, and time are measured on ratio scales. A person's weight, for instance, is measured on a ratio scale and it is acceptable to say that someone who weighs 200 lbs is twice as heavy as someone who weights 100 lbs. Ratio scales are commonly used in the health sciences (e.g., blood pressure, pulse). As we all know, however, temperature is not measured on a ratio scale in health care. If it was, the normal body temperature of humans would be 309.9° K.

THE VALUE OF MEASUREMENT

Although measurement is important in everyday life, it is particularly important in health care. Since measurement is based on explicit rules, it is objective and the values obtained on different measurement scales can be independently verified by anyone who uses the same measures. The hierarchy of scales also provides the ability to obtain greater and greater levels of precision in measurement. This precision facilitates communication. Rather than saying that a patient's blood pressure is high or his/her pulse is fast, one can state the exact blood pressure or pulse, which leaves no ambiguity (Polit & Hungler, 1989).

Measurement may be even more important in health care research because it provides a means to examine the relationships among disease risk factors and health outcomes. The degree of precision that can be achieved by such comparisons depends upon the level of measurement applied to the variables of interest (Dawson-Saunders & Trappan, 1994). With nominal scales, one can measure the frequency with which cases fall into different categories and obtain proportions. Thus, one can, for example, measure the most common symptoms of a given disease or the most common diseases in a population. With ordinal scales, one can rank the same symptoms or diseases in terms of their relative occurrence. Interval scales can be used to more closely assess the characteristics of the diseases, the symptoms themselves, and their relationship to risk and protective factors. Finally, the use of ratio scales allow researchers to measure both the incidence and prevalence of symptoms and diseases and their odds ratios, with respect to risk factors and protective factors. Each level of measurement enables crucial information to be communicated, thereby, improving research and practice in health care.

REFERENCES

Bailey, K. D. (1987). *Methods of social research* (3rd Ed.). New York, NY: The Free Press.

Beder, J., & Yan, G. W. (2013). VHA Chaplains: challenges, roles, rewards, and frustrations of the work. *Journal of Health Care Chaplaincy, 19*(2), 54–65.

Besterman-Dahan, K., Barnett, S., Hickling, E., Elnitsky, C., Lind, J., Skvoretz, J., & Antinori, N. (2012). Bearing the burden: Deployment stress among army National Guard chaplains. *Journal of Health Care Chaplaincy, 18*(3–4), 151–168.

Bridgman, P. W. (1927). *The logic of modern physics.* New York, NY: Macmillan.

Bridgman, P. W. (1938). Operational analysis. *Philosophy of Science, 5*(2), 114–131.

Bridgman, P. W. (1945). Some general principles of operational analysis. *Psychological Review, 52*(5), 246–249.

Dawson-Saunders, B., & Trappan, R. G. (1994). *Basic and clinical biostatistics* (2nd Ed.). Norwalk, CT: Appleton & Lange.

Ellis, L. (1998). *Research methods in the social sciences.* New York, NY: McGraw-Hill.

Kerlinger, F. N. (1973). *Foundations of behavioral research* (2nd Ed.). New York, NY: Holt, Rhinehart & Winston.

Polit, D. F., & Hungler, B. P. (1989). *Essentials of nursing research: Methods, appraisal, and utilization* (2nd Ed.). Philadelphia, PA: Lippincott.

Rubinson, L., & Neutens, J. J. (1987). *Research techniques in the health sciences.* New York, NY: Macmillan.

Stevens, S. S. (1935). The operational definition of psychological concepts. *Psychological Review, 42*(6), 517–527.

Stevens, S. S. (1946). On the theory of scales of measurement. *Science, 103*(2684), 677–680.

Stevens, S. S. (1975). *Psychophysics.* New York, NY: John Wiley.

Vanderwerker, L. C., Flannelly, K. J., Galek, K., Harding, S. R., Handzo, G. F., Oettinger, M., & Bauman, J. P. (2008). What do chaplains really do? III. Referrals in the New York Chaplaincy Study. *Journal of Health Care Chaplaincy, 14*(1), 57–73.

Vanderwerker, L. C., Handzo, G. F., Fogg, S. L., & Overvold, J. A. (2008). Selected findings from the "New York" and the "Metropolitan" chaplaincy studies: A 10-year comparison of chaplaincy in the New York City area. *Journal of Health Care Chaplaincy, 15*(1), 13–24.

Operational Definitions in Research on Religion and Health

KEVIN J. FLANNELLY, KATHERINE R. B. JANKOWSKI, and
LAURA T. FLANNELLY

This article summarizes the historical development of operational definitions and discusses their application to research on religion and health, and their importance for research, in general. The diversity of religious concepts that have been operationalized is described, as well as the development of multi-dimensional self-report measures of religion specifically designed for use in health research. The operational definitions of a variety of health concepts are also described, including the development of multi-dimensional self-report measures of health. Some of the most consistently observed salutary relationships between religion and health are mentioned. The rising interest in spirituality in health research is discussed, along with problems with the current operational definitions of spirituality in healthcare research. The levels of measurement used in various, operationally defined religious and healthcare concepts are highlighted.

The American physicist Percy Williams Bridgman introduced the term operational analysis in his 1927 book, *The Logic of Logic on Modern Physics* (Bridgman, 1927). Operational analysis refers to the process of defining scientific concepts by enumerating the procedures used to measure them. In essence, he said, a "concept is synonymous with a corresponding set of operations" (Bridgman, 1927, p. 5). He later conceded that he had oversimplified the point, and that a given set of operations may only capture one dimension of a multi-dimensional concept (Bridgman, 1938). Nevertheless, he argued, such definitions (which came to be called operational definitions; Crissman, 1939; Stevens, 1935) are necessary for science even if they do not sufficiently characterize the essence of a concept or construct.

Bridgman's idea of defining physical concepts by the operations used to measure them was inspired by his recognition of the degree to which Albert Einstein's theory of relativity had altered traditional ideas about physical concepts, including time and space. Hence, Bridgman's intent was to redefine scientific constructs empirically, and he questioned whether seemingly identical concepts that were measured by different methods were really the same thing. One can, for example, measure distance with a tape measure. However, this becomes impractical when distances are very large. As a result, surveyors use a theodolite, which does not measure distance, per se, but angles and the time it takes light to travel between two points. To Bridgman, distance measured in these two different ways, is not one concept, but two: *tape-measure distance*, and *theodolite distance*. Although this may seem to be an esoteric point, it is critical to know how a concept is measured in scientific research in any field of study.

The application of operational definitions to psychological concepts began in the 1930s (Crissman, 1939; Stevens, 1935), and there was extensive debate about the value and propriety of operational definitions in psychology in the 1930s and 1940s (e.g., Israel & Goldstein, 1944; McGregor, 1935). Some psychologists expressed concern that strictly adhering to Bridgman's principle would create new concepts for every way in which a concept might be measured (e.g., Waters & Pennington, 1938). However, the goal of operational definitions is not to create new concepts, but to inform people about the specific manner in which a concept is measured, so that they can judge for themselves if the operational definition is consistent with the generally accepted definition of the concept. One can thereby assess whether the methods used to measure the concept provide an adequate and valid measure of that concept.

SIMPLE OPERATIONAL DEFINITIONS OF RELIGION AND HEALTH

Imagine that you just read a newspaper story that stated, "Researchers find religion is good for your health." Given what we have said about operational definitions, what would be the first two questions you, or any researcher, should ask? In no particular order, the questions we would ask are: "How did they define religion?" and "How did they define health?" Or, given that operational definitions are all about measurement, those questions could just as well be stated as: "How did they measure religion?" and "How did they measure health?"

Early studies on the relationship between religion and health were not actually studies about religion and health, they were, in the words of Levin and Schiller (1987, p. 13), health surveys "in which religion ... made only rare 'guest appearances'." The guest appearances usually entailed a single survey question in which religion was often operationally defined as religious affiliation or denomination.[1] Levin and Schiller reviewed a number of studies in which religious denomination was associated with morbidity (i.e., disease) and mortality (i.e., death).[2]

Several early studies on religious affiliation and health compared the health of different religious denominations in terms of cause of death, which is easy to operationally define from death certificates, (Levin & Schiller, 1987). These and later studies have found, for example, that Jews, Mormons, and Seventh Day Adventists are less likely to die from heart disease than members of other religious denominations in the U.S. (Koenig, McCullough, & Larson, 2001).

Other research reported denominational differences in morbidity (Levin & Vanderpool, 1989). Mormons and Seventh-Day Adventists, for instance, also are less likely to have hypertension (i.e., high blood pressure[3]), which can lead to heart disease. Subsequent studies have confirmed these findings and other denominational differences in health outcomes (Koenig et al., 2001). Such denominational differences in mortality and morbidity probably reflect the effects of religious prohibitions against certain unhealthy behaviors (Ellison & Levin, 1998; Hummer, Ellison, Rogers, Moulton, & Romero, 2004).

In the 1960s, U.S. health researchers began to measure how often people attended religious services (Levin & Vanderpool, 1987). This was usually measured by simply asking "How often do you attend Sunday worship services"[4] (Hall, Meador, & Koenig, 2008, p. 140). Thus, the operational definition of religion in these studies was how often people attended weekly worship services on Sunday. Obviously, this operational definition excludes people who belong to religious faiths that do not regularly hold religious services on Sundays. However, the operational definition could be made more inclusive if it asked "How often do you attend weekly worship services." The advantage of defining religion this way, instead of religious denomination is that it provides (a) a behavioral measure of religious commitment rather than nominal membership, and (b) it can be used across religious denominations in which religious services are regularly practiced. As attendance is reported by individuals, rather than directly observed, however, the accuracy of answers to questions about religious attendance has been challenged (Flannelly, Ellison, & Strock, 2004).

Despite its limitations, self-reported attendance at religious services is the most widely used measure of religion in research on religion and health in the United States (Hall et al., 2008). Regularly attending religious services, regardless of religious denomination, is inversely related to hypertension (Levin & Vanderpool, 1989) and various other diseases that are more difficult to operationally define. Moreover, one of the most consistent findings in this research field is that people who frequently attend religious services are more likely to live longer (Hummer et al., 2004); an operationally simple, yet fairly comprehensive definition of heath. One must keep in mind, however, that regularly attending religious services may be associated with other aspects of aging that are associated with health and longevity, including physical mobility (Hummer et al., 2004).

COMPLEX OPERATIONAL DEFINITIONS
OF RELIGION AND HEALTH

Hill and Hood (1999) compiled a comprehensive collection of more than 100 scales of religion that typically consist of 25–50 questions, or items.[5] The scales measure various dimensions of religion, most of which are described as falling into the following categories: religious attitudes, beliefs, concerns, commitment, coping, doubts, experiences, expression, fundamentalism, ideology, internalization, involvement, maturity, practices, problem-solving, values, and well-being. Therefore, if you asked the question: "How did they define religion?" you could get over a 100 different answers. However, not many of these scales were useful for research on religion and health, partly because of their length, so the Fetzer Institute assembled a team of researchers to develop scales that would be more useful (Fetzer Institute, 1999).

The Fetzer team developed a dozen scales, most of which have short versions of 2–6 items to make them easy to use in healthcare research (Fetzer Institute, 1999).[6] Nine separate scales operationally define religious beliefs, commitment, coping, history (like a medical history), preference (i.e., denomination), support (from congregants), and values, as well as private religious practices (such as prayer), and "organizational religiousness" (such as attending services). Three other scales were developed to measure forgiveness, meaning, and daily spiritual experiences. Finally, the group put together a 38-item multi-dimensional scale that contains all 12 of these dimensions, along with an overall self-rating of religiousness: To what extent do you consider yourself a religious person?

Hall et al. (2008) provide a comprehensive review of religious measures, in which they recommend some other useful scales. They also provide a critique of the interpretation and value of different types of religious measures used in healthcare research. They are skeptical, for instance, of global self-assessments of religiousness, such as the single question asked in the Fetzer scale, because of their inherent subjectivity.

Interest in spirituality rose substantially among healthcare researchers in the 1980s and 1990s and it surged near the end of the twentieth century (Weaver, Flannelly, & Oppenheimer, 2003; Weaver, Pargament, Flannelly, & Oppenheimer, 2006). The rising interest in spirituality coincided with a change in the definition of spirituality, from being an aspect of religion to being something separate from religion, especially organized religion (Hill & Pargament, 2003). Since the turn of the century, numerous scales of spirituality have been developed and used in health research.

Koenig, however, has expressed concerns about the operational definitions of spirituality in health research. Koenig and his colleagues (Koenig, 2008; Koenig et al., 2001) say most scales of spirituality are operationally defined in terms of positive emotional states and not in terms of anything that is distinctly spiritual or religious. In the Fetzer Institute's scale of daily spiritual experiences, for example, close to half of the questions are about acceptance, caring, compassion, harmony, gratitude, mercy, and peace (Fetzer Institute, 1999). Many other spirituality scales used in health research operationally define spirituality, at least in part, as feelings of peace and harmony, a sense of meaning and purpose in life, and other positive emotions (e.g., Monod et al., 2011). Yet, research outside the United States indicates that the concept of spirituality defined by positive attitudes and feelings is only one of six dimensions of spirituality (la Cour & Gotke, 2012).

Operationally defining spirituality in terms of positive emotions is particularly troubling for interpreting reports of beneficial associations between spirituality and mental health (Koenig, 2008). What does it mean, for example, when a study reports an inverse association between spirituality and depression? As depressed individuals often lack feelings of peace and harmony or a sense of meaning and purpose in life, depressed people will score low on spirituality. The predictor variable (spirituality) is contaminated with the outcome variable (depression); therefore, a reported result of an inverse association between spirituality and depression is tautological: people who have feelings of peace and harmony and/or a sense of meaning and purpose in life are not depressed.

Koenig (2008) makes another, equally important, point about interpreting the results of studies reporting beneficial associations between spirituality and health. As positive psychological well-being appears to have a beneficial effect on physical health (e.g., Ellison & Levin, 1998), measures that define spirituality in terms of psychological well-being conflate the effects of spirituality with the effects of psychological well-being on physical health. Research is needed to operationally define spirituality as distinctly different from positive emotions.

The International Statistical Classification of Diseases and Related Health Problems (ICD for short) lists well over 1,000 diseases and physical and mental disorders. Therefore, if you asked the question, "How did they define health?" you could get a thousand or more different answers. However, only a small subset of these health problems has attracted the attention of researchers interested in the relationship between religion and health, according to the *Handbook of Religion and Health* (Koenig et al., 2001). Unfortunately, for our purposes, the *Handbook* is better at identifying the operational definitions of religion than the operational definitions of health.

Although the operational definitions of mental disorders are complex, they usually are based on responses to a series of questions that capture the diagnostic criteria of a disorder (*DSM IV-TR*, 2000). Scales based on validated operational definitions of various mental disorders are freely available, including some that may be particularly useful in chaplaincy research, such as measures of anxiety (Spitzer, Kroenke, Williams, & Lowe, 2006) and depression (Kroenke, Spitzer, & Williams, 2001).

Two of the mostly frequently studied diseases listed in the *Handbook* are cancer and heart disease. As these are very broad categories of disease, we will mention only a few examples of their operational definitions. A selective review of the literature on religion and health indicated that cancer is often operationally defined by site (or type of cancer) and stage[7] (e.g., Hebert, Zdaniuk, Schulz, & Scheier, 2009; Kune, Kune, & Watson, 1993; Nelson et al., 2009). Many other studies have examined the relationship between religion and cancer mortality or operationally defined risk factors (Koenig et al., 2001) or symptoms (e.g., Bekelman et al., 2009). Although some earlier studies found that religion was a protective factor for cancer (e.g., Kune et al., 1993), recent research has focused on the association between religious coping and subjective measures of patient well-being and quality of life (e.g., Hebert et al., 2009; Nelson et al., 2009).

Religion has been found to have a salubrious association with several types of heart diseases, or heart disorders (Koenig et al., 2001),[8] and with risk factors for some heart disorders, including levels[9] of interferon gamma and anti-inflammatory cytokines (Lucchese & Koenig, 2013). Since the publication of the *Handbook* (Koenig et al., 2001), more than 20 studies have examined the relationship between some measure of religion (often prayer) and health outcomes following heart surgery. The operationally defined physical health outcomes have included post-operative length of stay, infections, other complications, and cardiac functioning, such as the Left Ventricular Ejection Fraction[10] (Ai et al., 2010; Mouch & Sonnega, 2012).

Although surveys have been used in epidemiology for many years, the 1986–1987 Medical Outcomes Study (MOS) was the first major U.S. study to survey out-patients about their health (Tarlov et al., 1989). To do this, the RAND corporation developed the MOS 36-Item Short-Form Health Survey, more commonly known as the SF-36 (Ware & Sherbourne, 1992).[11] The SF-36, which is still widely used, measures eight operationally defined dimensions of health: physical functioning, role limitations caused by physical problems, bodily pain, general health, vitality, social functioning, role limitations caused by emotional problems, and mental health. The SF-36, which was validated with clinical data (McHorney, Ware, & Raczek, 1993), is often used as the sole measure of health status in many studies.

The success of the SF-36 spurred the development of many other patient self-report measures of physical health that are widely used in all areas of health research, including research on religion and health. Some researchers adapted the SF-36 and others created a variety of scales that are generally referred to as quality of life measures. A number of these instruments have been developed to measure patients' symptoms and psychological adjustment to specific diseases, including kidney disease and different types of cancer.

OPERATIONAL DEFINITIONS AND CHAPLAINCY

It is particularly important to be clear about the operational definitions of what one is discussing and measuring. This is as important in the everyday practice of chaplains as it is for other health professionals. The words a chaplain uses to define what occurred during a pastoral visit with a patient, and the words that are written in a chart determine the clarity of understanding about what occurred during the visit, and the relationship between what occurred during the visit and patient outcomes. What is presence, healing touch, prayer, or even a religious discussion with a patient? Are these behaviors best defined by the chaplain alone? It is possible that patients will have insight into defining these things, so chaplains might consider collaborating with patients in defining these and other concepts? We know that chaplaincy research is not considered to be a burden by some patients (Winter-Pfandler & Morgenthaler, 2010), and some patients may be eager to participate in research. In conclusion, while operationally defining a concept can be a distinctly difficult task, operational definitions are essential in research because by making concepts explicit they enhance understanding.

NOTES

1. Religious denomination represents a nominal level of measurement, or nominal scale, in which a variable is classified into categories that have no real numerical value.

2. Their review covered studies published between 1837 and 1984.

3. Hypertension represents a nominal level of measurement, because it is the name for a, or category of disease. Blood pressure, itself, is measured on a ratio scale.

4. Frequency of attending religious services is technically a ratio scale because some people never attend religious services, but it is usually treated as an interval scale for methodological reasons.

5. The items on most of the scales are measured by ratings that are assumed to represent equal intervals, which are summed to form a total score for the scale.

6. As of this writing, the Fetzer report, which include all of the scales, could be downloaded for free at https://www.gem-beta.org/public/MeasureDetail.aspx?mid=1155&cat=2

7. Cancer site, or type of cancer (colon, breast, throat, etc.), is another example of a nominal scale. The stages of cancer are ranked on an ordinal scale, in which higher numbers (e.g., I, II, III, and IV) represent greater progression and severity of disease.

8. Heart disease is classified on a nominal scale into several diseases or disorders: arrhythmias, cardiomyopathy, conduction, congenital, coronary artery, hypertensive, infective, rheumatic, valvular, and congestive heart failure.

9. Levels of interferon gamma and anti-inflammatory cytokines are measured on ratio scales in which there are equal intervals and a meaningful zero point; zero means they are not present.

10. The Left Ventricular Ejection Fraction is the volume of blood pumped out of the ventricle with each heartbeat.

11. The SF-36 can be downloaded for free from the RAND Corporation, as the RAND 36-Item Health Survey.

REFERENCES

Ai, A. L., Ladd, K. L., Peterson, C., Cook, C. A., Shearer, M., & Koenig, H. G. (2010). Long-term adjustment after surviving open heart surgery: The effect of using prayer for coping replicated in a prospective design. *Gerontologist, 50*(6), 798–809.

Bekelman, D. B., Rumsfeld, J. S., Havranek, E. P., Yamashita, T. E., Hutt, E., Gottlieb, S. H., . . . , Kutner, J. S. (2009). Symptom burden, depression, and spiritual well-being: A comparison of heart failure and advanced cancer patients. *Journal of General and Internal Medicine, 24*(5), 592–598.

Bridgman, P. W. (1927). *The logic of modern physics.* New York, NY: Macmillan.

Bridgman, P. W. (1938). Operational analysis. *Philosophy of Science, 5*(2), 114–131.

Crissman, P. (1939). The operational definition of concepts. *Psychological Review, 46*(4), 309–317.

Diagnostic & Statistical Manual of Mental Disorders (Text Revision) (DSM IV-TR). (2000). Washington, DC: American Psychiatric Association.

Ellison, C. G., & Levin, J. S. (1998). The religion-health connection: Evidence, theory and future directions. *Health Education & Behavior, 25*16(700–720).

Fetzer Institute. (1999). *Multidimensional measurement of religiousness/spirituality for use in health research.* Kalamazoo, MI: John E. Fetzer Institute.

Flannelly, K., Ellison, C., & Strock, A. (2004). Methodologic issues in research on religion and health. *Southern Medical Journal, 97*(12), 1231–1241.

Hall, D. E., Meador, K. G., & Koenig, H. G. (2008). Measuring religiousness in and health research. *Journal of Religion & Health, 47,* 134–183.

Hebert, R., Zdaniuk, B., Schulz, R., & Scheier, M. (2009). Positive and negative religious coping and well-being in women with breast cancer. *Journal of Palliative Medicine, 12*(6), 537–545.

Hill, P., & Pargament, K. (2003). Advances in the conceptualization and measurement of religion and spirituality. *American Psychologist, 58*(1), 64–74.

Hill, P. C., & Hood Jr., R. W. (Eds.). (1999). *Measures of religiosity.* Birmingham, AL: Religious Education Press.

Hummer, R. A., Ellison, C. G., Rogers, R. G., Moulton, B. E., & Romero, R. R. (2004). Religious involvement and adult mortality in the United States: Review and perspectives. *Southern Medical Journal, 97*(12), 1223–1230.

Israel, H., & Goldstein, B. (1944). Operationism in psychology. *Psychological Review, 51*(3), 177–188.

Koenig, H. G. (2008). Concerns about measuring "spirituality" in research. *Journal of Nervous and Mental Disease, 196*(5), 349–355.

Koenig, H. G., McCullough, M. E., & Larson, D. B. (2001). *Handbook of religion and health.* New York, NY: Oxford University Press.

Kroenke, K., Spitzer, R. L., & Williams, J. B. (2001). The PHQ-9: Validity of a brief depression severity measure. *Journal of General and Internal Medicine, 16*(9), 606–613.

Kune, G. A., Kune, S., & Watson, L. F. (1993). Perceived religiousness is protective for colorectal cancer: Data from the Melbourne Colorectal Cancer Study. *Journal of the Royal Society of Medicine, 86*(11), 645–647.

la Cour, P., & Gotke, P. (2012). Understanding of the word "spirituality" by theologians compared to lay people: An empirical study from a secular region. *Journal of Health Care Chaplaincy, 18*(3–4), 97–109.

Levin, J. S., & Schiller, P. L. (1987). Is there a religious factor in health? *Journal of Religion & Health, 26*(1), 9–36.

Levin, J. S., & Vanderpool, H. Y. (1987). Is frequent religious attendance really conducive to better health? Toward an epidemiology of religion. *Social Science & Medicine, 24*(7), 589–600.

Levin, J. S., & Vanderpool, H. Y. (1989). Is religion therapeutically significant for hypertension? *Social Science & Medicine, 29*(1), 69–78.

Lucchese, F. A., & Koenig, H. G. (2013). Religion, spirituality and cardiovascular disease: Research, clinical implications, and opportunities in Brazil. *Revista Brasileira de Cirurgia Cardiovascular, 28*(1), 103–128.

McGregor, D. (1935). Scientific measurement and psychology. *Psychological Review, 42*(3), 246–266.

McHorney, C. A., Ware, J. E., Jr., & Raczek, A. E. (1993). The MOS 36-Item Short-Form Health Survey (SF-36): II. Psychometric and clinical tests of validity in measuring physical and mental health constructs. *Medical Care, 31*(3), 247–263.

Monod, S., Brennan, M., Rochat, E., Martin, E., Rochat, S., & Bula, C. J. (2011). Instruments measuring spirituality in clinical research: A systematic review. *Journal of General and Internal Medicine, 26*(11), 1345–1357.

Mouch, C. A., & Sonnega, A. J. (2012). Spirituality and recovery from cardiac surgery: A review. *Journal of Religion and Health, 51*(4), 1042–1060.

Nelson, C., Jacobson, C. M., Weinberger, M. I., Bhaskaran, V., Rosenfeld, B., Breitbart, W., & Roth, A. J. (2009). The role of spirituality in the relationship between religiosity and depression in prostate cancer patients. *Annals of Behavioral Medicine, 38*(2), 105–114.

Spitzer, R. L., Kroenke, K., Williams, J. B., & Lowe, B. (2006). A brief measure for assessing generalized anxiety disorder: The GAD-7. *Archives of Internal Medicine, 166*(10), 1092–1097.

Stevens, S. S. (1935). The operational definition of psychological concepts. *Psychological Review, 42*(6), 517–527.

Tarlov, A. R., Ware, J. E., Jr., Greenfield, S., Nelson, E. C., Perrin, E., & Zubkoff, M. (1989). The Medical Outcomes Study. An application of methods for monitoring the results of medical care. *Journal of the American Medical Association, 262*(7), 925–930.

Ware, J. E., Jr., & Sherbourne, C. D. (1992). The MOS 36-item short-form health survey (SF-36). I. Conceptual framework and item selection. *Medical Care, 30*(6), 473–483.

Waters, R. H., & Pennington, L. A. (1938). Operationism in psychology. *Psychological Review, 45*(5), 414–423.

Weaver, A. J., Flannelly, K. J., & Oppenheimer, B. A. (2003). Religion, spirituality, and chaplains in the biomedical literature: 1965–2000. *International Journal of Psychiatry in Medicine, 33*(2), 155–161.

Weaver, A. J., Pargament, K. I., Flannelly, K. J., & Oppenheimer, J. E. (2006). Trends in the scientific study of religion, spirituality, and health: 1965–2000. *Journal of Religion and Health, 45*(2), 208–214.

Winter-Pfandler, U., & Morgenthaler, C. (2010). Are surveys on quality improvement of healthcare chaplaincy emotionally distressing for patients? A pilot study. *Journal of Health Care Chaplaincy, 16*(3–4), 140–148.

Independent, Dependent, and Other Variables in Healthcare and Chaplaincy Research

LAURA T. FLANNELLY,KEVINJ.FLANNELLYand
KATHERINE R. B. JANKOWSKI

This article begins by defining the term variable and the terms independent variable and dependent variable, providing examples of each. It then proceeds to describe and discuss synonyms for the terms independent variable and dependent variable, including treatment, intervention, predictor, and risk factor, and synonyms for dependent variable, such as response variables and outcomes. The article explains that the terms extraneous, nuisance, and confounding variables refer to any variable that can interfere with the ability to establish relationships between independent variables and dependent variables, and it describes ways to control for such confounds. It further explains that even though intervening, mediating, and moderating variables explicitly alter the relationship between independent variables and dependent variables, they help to explain the causal relationship between them. In addition, the article links terminology about variables with the concept of levels of measurement in research.

Anyone who wants to understand healthcare research should start by learning research terminology. The term *variable* is probably the most frequently used word in scientific research. However, people who have not been trained in research often find the word to be odd. The simplest definition of a variable is that it is something that takes on different values; it is something that varies (Bhopal, 2002; Kerlinger, 1973). Within the context of research, a variable may be defined as "an empirical phenomenon that takes on different values or intensities" (Ellis, 1998, p. 19).

A variable also may be thought of as a property of something (Kerlinger, 1973). The height, weight, and temperature of an object are three examples of its properties. Human research measures, among other things, the properties of people. These properties may include their height, weight, and temperature, as well as other properties (i.e., variables), such as, intelligence, personality, and health status.

Variables are generally divided into two broad categories in research, *independent* variables and *dependent* variables. However, researchers refer to them by many different names, and there are other types of variables, as well.

INDEPENDENT AND DEPENDENT VARIABLES

Most healthcare professionals have heard the terms independent variable and dependent variable (Kleinbaum, Kupper, Muller, & Nizam, 1998; Polit, Beck, & Hungler, 2001), but they may not know what they mean or know the difference between them. Although the terms are similar, their meanings are very different, and the ability to distinguish between the two of them is essential for understanding and designing research studies.

One of the major aims of research is to understand the causes of phenomena. The presumed cause in a cause-effect relationship is called the independent variable, and the presumed effect is called the dependent variable (Polit et al., 2001; Vogt, 1993). In other words, an independent variable is a variable that is presumed to have an effect on another variable (a dependent variable). A dependent variable is, quite simply, dependent, in that it depends, in some sense, on an independent variable. It is the dependent variable that the researcher is usually most interested in understanding and possibly interested in predicting.

It is important to remember, however, that variables are not inherently independent or dependent variables. An independent variable in one study might be a dependent variable in another study. For example, one study might examine the effect of exercise (the independent variable) on osteoporosis (the dependent variable); another study might examine the effect of osteoporosis (the independent variable) on the occurrence of bone fractures (the dependent variable).

The use of the term independent variable arose in the context of experimentation, and the purpose of most experiments is to test whether an independent variable, in fact, does have an effect on one or more dependent variables. A simple experiment might test whether exercise (the independent variable) has an effect on body weight (the dependent variable) by having people engage in physical exercise for different amounts of time. Many experiments in healthcare are referred to as randomized control trials (RCTs). An example of an RCT is a study in which individuals are randomly assigned to groups that exercise for different amounts of time to see if exercise has an effect on body weight. Another example of an RCT is a study that randomly assigns individuals to several groups that receive different doses of a diuretic (the independent variable) to test whether diuretics have an effect on blood pressure (the dependent variable). Many types of medical treatments have been examined as independent variables in RCTs to evaluate their effects on a predetermined health outcome (the dependent variable). An independent variable in an RCT can be as simple as a drug dosage, or as complex as a surgical procedure, or a series of medical treatments, such as chemotherapy.

An example that readers of the *Journal of Health Care Chaplaincy* will be familiar with is an RCT by Toussaint, Barry, Bornfriend, and Markman (2014), in which they randomly assigned patients to two conditions, or groups. The experimental group engaged in educational activities related to forgiveness (their independent variable), while the control group did not. The study tested whether the independent variable of educational activities had an effect on a number of dependent variables, including pessimism, self-acceptance, and self-forgiveness. The independent variable only had an effect on self-forgiveness. As often happens, the authors did not use the terms independent variable or dependent variable, and, therefore, readers had to figure them out for themselves.

Although the independent variable is not manipulated in nonexperimental research, the term independent variable is widely used in nonexperimental studies. For example, Galek et al. (2010) were explicit about what their independent and dependent variables were in a study of whether a chaplain's gender or religious affiliation influenced praying with patients. The independent variables were not limited to the gender and religious denomination of the chaplains; they also included whether the gender and denominations of the chaplains were the same as the gender and denominations of the patients they visited. The dependent variable was simply the percentage of visits in which chaplains prayed with patients. A key finding of the study was that chaplains were more likely to pray with patients from their own religion. It should be mentioned that personal or demographic characteristics are often treated as independent variables in experimental and nonexperimental studies.

TREATMENTS, INTERVENTIONS, AND OUTCOMES

Some researchers only use the term independent variable in the context of experimental research, and some researchers do not use the term, even when reporting an experiment or RCT. This is particularly true in healthcare research where the terms *treatment* and *intervention* often are used instead of independent variable. Likewise, many researchers prefer to use the term, *outcome* in favor of dependent variable. Montonye and Calderone (2009), for example, use the terms intervention and outcomes, instead of independent and dependent variables, in an observational study of specific chaplain interventions to address patients' feelings, attitudes, and issues.

One of the few experimental studies of chaplaincy used the words treatment and intervention, instead of independent variable, when referring to chaplain visits with patients. The study also used the word outcomes instead of dependent variables when referring to the effects of chaplain visits on patient anxiety, depression, hope, and coping (Bay, Beckman, Trippi, Gunderman, & Terry, 2008). The chaplain intervention only had an effect on negative religious coping. It is worth noting here that the term "effect" typically is used only when a causal relationship between an intervention and an outcome (i.e., independent variable and dependent variable) can be demonstrated experimentally. Therefore, the term effect typically is not used in reference to nonexperimental studies, as those studies only describe the associations or relationships between variables.

PREDICTOR, RESPONSE, AND MORE OUTCOME VARIABLES

The term *predictor* often is used in nonexperimental research (Kleinbaum et al., 1998) to refer to a variable that can predict another variable i.e., the magnitude of the predictor (independent variable) can predict the magnitude of another variable (dependent variable). The term predictor is useful because it does not imply that the predictor causes the change in the predicted variable, although it may. Grossoehme, Szczesniak, McPhail, and Seid (2013) examined the association between religious coping in adolescents with cystic fibrosis and the rate of change in their pulmonary function. Their *predictor* (or independent variable) was pulmonary functioning, which predicted the subsequent religious coping by the adolescents. The authors referred to religious coping as a *response variable*, which is another name for a dependent variable (Kleinbaum et al., 1998).

A cross-sectional survey by Gaudette and Jankowski (2013) on the associations of religious beliefs and spiritual practices with anxiety in palliative-care patients used the terms independent and predictor variable interchangeably when referring to beliefs and spiritual practices. The study found that both of the independent variables predicted anxiety. They also used the term outcomes when discussing the results of previous research, but described anxiety as their dependent variable.

A cross-sectional survey of physicians provides another example of the use of the terms predictors and outcomes (King, Dimmers, Langer & Murphy,

2013). One of the study's key findings was that greater knowledge of chaplains predicted the extent to which the physicians tried to address spirituality in their care of patients, and to refer patients to spiritual care providers.

RISK FACTORS AND PROTECTIVE FACTORS

Many healthcare researchers, especially epidemiologists, use the term risk factor when referring to what otherwise would be called an independent variable (Kelsey, Thompson, & Evans, 1986; Kleinbaum, Kupper, & Morgenstern, 1982). There are at least two reasons for this. First, many diseases have multiple causes, as expressed in the notion of "the web of causation" (Kelsey et al., 1986, p. 33). Second, it is difficult to establish causality in nonexperimental research (see K. J. Flannelly & Jankowski, 2014). The use of the general term, risk factor, avoids the question of causality. The Framingham Heart Study, which introduced the term "risk factor" (Berridge, Gorsky, & Mold, 2011) found that high levels of blood cholesterol, high blood pressure, obesity, cigarette smoking, and age were key risk factors for coronary heart disease, in that they increased the risk of having the disease (Kannel, Dawber, Kagan, Revotskie, & Stokes, 1961).

Variables that reduce the risk of disease are called protective factors. Numerous studies, for example, have found that having a religious affiliation (i.e., belonging to a religious denomination) is a protective factor for heart disease (Koenig, McCullough, & Larson, 2001).

EXTRANEOUS, NUISANCE, OR CONFOUNDING VARIABLES

Another type of variable to be aware of when reading or designing studies goes by many different names, including extraneous variable, nuisance variable, and confounding variable, or simply confound or confounder (Kleinbaum et al., 1982; 1998; Polit et al., 2001). Researchers are concerned about extraneous variables because they can alter or obscure the relationship between the independent variable and dependent variable, or indicate there is a causal relationship between them when none exists. Researchers try to control for extraneous variables in their experiments by controlling the conditions of the experimental environment to keep variables as constant as possible (Polit et al., 2001). In human research however, experimental control often is not sufficient because individuals vary in many ways that are extraneous to the purpose of a study. Such extraneous variables may include their age, gender, ethnicity, income, and education. If experimental control is not possible, the researcher has three options for dealing with extraneous variables (Polit et al., 2001). One way is to try to match the study participants on the possible confounds, such as matching experimental and control subjects, or cases and noncases, by age, gender, and other key possible confounding variables. However, this can be difficult to do. Another way is to incorporate an extraneous variable as an independent variable in the study design. If age, for example, might have an effect on the relationship between the independent variable and dependent variable, the researcher can group participants into subgroups of different ages, say, 20 year-olds, 30 year-olds, 40 year-olds, and so forth. This method is called "stratification," and the "effects" of stratified variables are usually included in the statistical analyses (Mausner & Kramer, 1985). The third way is to use the person's age as an independent variable in the statistical analyses. It is a common practice to measure an extraneous variable and include the measure of it only in the statistical analysis as a way to control for variation in the levels of the variable among the study's participants. This practice is particularly common in survey studies. Regardless of the approach used to control extraneous variables, it is always important to see if the participants vary in ways that could affect the dependent variable.

When extraneous variables are used as independent variables in the statistical analyses, they are called covariates. Demographic and other personal characteristics are considered to be covariates (i.e., controls) or independent variables in statistical analyses contingent upon whether a researcher is specifically interested in the relationship between these variables and the dependent variable(s). Studies on the relationship between religion and health should, and usually do, statistically control for age, gender, and ethnicity because these variables are associated with variation in the level of religious involvement, practices, and other expressions of religious faith (Flannelly, Ellison, & Strock, 2004).

INTERVENING, MEDIATING, AND MODERATING VARIABLES

There are three other terms that are used exclusively in reference to possible causal variables: intervening, mediating, and moderating variables. Tolman (1938) used the term intervening variable to refer to a variable or set of variables in a chain of causation in which the intervening variable is the causal link between the independent and dependent variable of interest. In his analysis of the concept, intervening variables are unobserved theoretical constructs, but the term can be applied just as well to observed variables. A major point of his paper is that the effect of an independent variable on a dependent variable can be demonstrated to occur through the causal chain of the independent, intervening, and dependent variables. Hence, an intervening variable is an independent variable in its own right. Today, such intervening variables are called mediating variables (Cohen, Cohen, West, & Aiken, 2003).

The well-established positive relationship between religion and health, often reflects, or at least implies, such a chain of causation. For example, numerous studies have found that people that have a religious affiliation are less likely to have heart disease, and this is especially true for people who belong to The Seventh-Day Adventist Church and The Church of Jesus Christ of Latter-Day Saints (Koenig et al., 2001). A closer look at the association between religious affiliation and heart disease reveals that people who belong to The Seventh-Day Adventist Church and The Church of Jesus Christ of Latter-Day Saints also are less likely to have hypertension (i.e., high blood pressure), which can lead to heart disease (Koenig et al., 2001). Thus, hypertension appears to mediate the positive association between religious affiliation and heart disease. We can extend the chain of causation to identify intervening variables that may mediate the connection between religious affiliation and reduced blood pressure.

Ellison and Levin (1998) present a comprehensive review of why denominational differences and other aspects of religion mediate the effects of religion on health. Some of these entail proscriptions against certain kinds of behavior, such as prohibitions against drinking alcohol and coffee by the Latter-Day Saints and Seventh-Day Adventist Churches, which are risk factors for hypertension. Other aspects of religious affiliation also mediate the relationship between religion and health, including the salutary effects of social support provided by religious congregations that reduce the stress associated with illness and disease (Ellison & Levin, 1998).

Moderating variables alter the strength of association (and possibly the direction of association) between independent and dependent variables (Cohen et al., 2003). A comparison of two related studies will help to demonstrate this point. Both studies analyzed survey data from the same sample of American adults. The first study examined the relationship between mental health and spiritual struggles, that is, feeling alienated from God (McConnell, Pargament, Ellison, & Flannelly, 2006). After statistically controlling for age, education, gender, income, race, social support, strength of religious identity, and the frequency of praying and attending religious services, McConnell et al. (2006) found, as hypothesized, that the spiritual struggles were associated with higher levels of anxiety and depression. While prayer also was positively related to anxiety and depression, the strength of religious identity and attending services were unrelated to either anxiety or depression. The second study hypothesized that the association of spiritual struggles with anxiety and depression would be moderated by the strength of a person's religious identity (Ellison, Fang, Flannelly, & Steckler, 2013), and this proved to be the case. Controlling for the same variables analyzed in the first study (McConnell et al., 2006), the second study found that strength of religious identity moderated the association between spiritual struggles and both anxiety and depression. That is, symptoms of depression and anxiety among individuals with spiritual struggles were higher for individuals who were more religious than for individuals who were less religious. By itself, strength of religious identity had no association with anxiety or depression, yet it moderated (in this case, aggravated) the adverse association between spiritual struggles and mental health (Ellison et al., 2013).

CATEGORICAL, DISCRETE, AND CONTINUOUS VARIABLES

All of the previous terms we have discussed thus far have to do with the relationship among variables. These three terms are not about the relation-ship among variables, but the measurement of variables. The first term, categorical variable, was defined and discussed by Flannelly, Flannelly, and Jankowski (2014) in an earlier paper in this series of articles on *Research Methodology*. Categorical variables present a nominal level of measurement, in which objects or people are classified into categories based on certain characteristics. People, for example, are often classified into categories by their gender, ethnicity, occupation, religious denomination, and, in the healthcare context, as either cases or noncases of disease.

Discrete variables are variables that have two or more values (Ellis, 1998). Hence, categorical variables technically are also discrete variables. It should be noted that variables that only have two values are called dichotomous variables.

More specifically, however, the term discrete refers to the fact that a variable is measured in whole numbers, whereas continuous variables may take on a virtually infinite number of values (Bailey, 1987; Indrayan, 2013). Many discrete variables are measured at the interval level of measurement, in which the points on the scale are separated by equal intervals, but there is no true zero point (see Flannelly et al., 2014). However, discrete variables may also be measured on ratio scales, which have a true zero point. Frequency measures, such as frequency of attending religious services or fre-quency of visiting a physician are good examples. Many healthcare variables are measured on ratios scales and are continuous variables, for example, age, weight, and blood levels of enzymes.

It is often the case that a variable that has an underlying continuum, may be measured as a discrete variable. For example, age is usually measured as a discrete variable, that is, years of age. It is also common to measure age as a categorical variable for example, infant, child, adolescent, and adult (Ellis, 1998). It is even common in healthcare research to measure age as a dichot-omous variable, such as, under 50 years of age, and 50 years of age and older.

SUMMARY

The present article was written to help readers unfamiliar with research terms to navigate their way through the maze of terminology used to describe the relationships among variables, as well as those used with respect to measuring variables. Anything that is measured in research is called a variable, and variables broadly fall into two categories: independent variables and dependent variables. The terms treatment, intervention, predictor, and risk factor are essentially synonyms for independent variable, and the terms response variable and outcomes are synonyms for dependent variable. As previously explained, extraneous, nuisance, and confounding variables are terms for a variable that can interfere with the ability to establish relationships between independent and dependent variables, and, therefore, different methods have been developed to control for them. On the other hand, although intervening, mediating, and moderating variables alter the relationship between independent and dependent variables, they help to explain the causal relationship between them. The final section tied together some terminology applied to the measurement of variables with the concept of levels of measurement in research.

REFERENCES

Bailey, K. D. (1987). *Methods of social research* (3rd ed.). New York, NY: The Free Press.

Bay, P. S., Beckman, D., Trippi, J., Gunderman, R., & Terry, C. (2008). The effect of pastoral care services on anxiety, depression, hope, religious coping, and religious problem solving styles: A randomized controlled study. *Journal of Religion and Health, 47*(1), 57–69.

Berridge, V., Gorsky, M., & Mold, A. (2011). *Public health in history.* Berkshire, UK: Open University Press.

Bhopal, R. S. (2002). *Concepts of epidemiology: An integrated introduction to the ideas, theories, principles and methods of epidemiology.* Oxford: Oxford University Press.

Cohen, J., Cohen, P., West, S. G., & Aiken, L. S. (2003). *Applied multiple regression/ correlation analyses for the behavioral sciences* (3rd ed.). Mahwah, NJ: Lawrence Erlbaum Associates.

Ellis, L. (1998). *Research methods in the social sciences.* New York, NY: McGraw-Hill.

Ellison, C. G., Fang, Q., Flannelly, K. J., & Steckler, R. A. (2013). Spiritual struggles and mental health: Exploring the moderating effects of religious identity. *International Journal for the Psychology of Religion, 23*(3), 214–229.

Ellison, C. G., & Levin, J. S. (1998). The religion-health connection: Evidence, theory and future directions. *Health Education & Behavior, 25*(6), 700–720.

Flannelly, K. J., Ellison, C. G., & Strock, A. L. (2004). Methodologic issues in research on religion and health. *Southern Medical Journal, 97*(12), 1231–1241.

Flannelly, K. J., & Jankowski, K. R. B. (2014). Research designs and making causal inferences from healthcare studies. *Journal of Health Care Chaplaincy, 20*(1), 23–38.

Flannelly, L. T., Flannelly, K. J., & Jankowski, K. R. B. (2014). Fundamentals of measurement in healthcare research. *Journal of Health Care Chaplaincy, 20*(2), 75–82.

Galek, K., Silton, N. R., Vanderwerker, L. C., Handzo, G. F., Porter, M., Montonye, M. G., & Fleenor, D. W. (2010). To pray or not to pray: Considering gender and religious concordance in praying with the ill. *Journal of Health Care Chaplaincy, 16*(1–2), 42–52.

Gaudette, H., & Jankowski, K. R. (2013). Spiritual coping and anxiety in palliative care patients: A pilot study. *Journal of Health Care Chaplaincy, 19*(4), 131–139.

Grossoehme, D. H., Szczesniak, R., McPhail, G. L., & Seid, M. (2013). Is Adolescents' religious coping with cystic fibrosis associated with the rate of decline in pulmonary function? – A preliminary study. *Journal of Health Care Chaplaincy, 19*(1), 33–42.

Indrayan, A. (2013). *Medical biostatistics* (3rd ed.). Boca Raton, FL: CRC Press.

Kannel, W. B., Dawber, T. R., Kagan, A., Revotskie, N., & Stokes, J. (1961). Factors of risk in the development of coronary heart disease—Six-year follow-up experience: The Framingham Study. *Annals of Internal Medicine, 55*(1), 33–50.

Kelsey, J., Thompson, W. D., & Evans, A. S. (1986). *Methods in observational epidemiology*. New York, NY: Oxford University Press.

Kerlinger, F. N. (1973). *Foundations of behavorial research* (2nd ed.). New York, NY: Holt, Rhinehart & Winston.

King, S. D., Dimmers, M. A., Langer, S., & Murphy, P. E. (2013). Doctors' attentiveness to the spirituality/religion of their patients in pediatric and oncology settings in the Northwest USA. *Journal of Health Care Chaplaincy, 19*(4), 140–164.

Kleinbaum, D. G., Kupper, L. L., & Morgenstern, H. (1982). *Epidemiologic research: Principles and quantitative methods*. New York, NY: Van Nostrand Reinhold.

Kleinbaum, D. G., Kupper, L. L., Muller, K. E., & Nizam, A. (1998). *Applied regression analysis and other multivariable methods*. Pacific Grove, CA: Duxbury Press.

Koenig, H. G., McCullough, M. E., & Larson, D. B. (2001). *Handbook of religion and health*. New York, NY: Oxford University Press.

Mausner, J., & Kramer, S. (1985). *Epidemiology: An introductory text (2nd ed.)*. Philadelphia, PA: W.P. Saunders.

McConnell, K. M., Pargament, K. I., Ellison, C. G., & Flannelly, K. J. (2006). Examining the links between spiritual struggles and symptoms of psychopathology in a national sample. *Journal of Clinical Psychology, 62*(12), 1469–1484.

Montonye, M., & Calderone, S. (2009). Pastoral interventions and the influence of self-reporting: A preliminary analysis. *Journal of Health Care Chaplaincy, 16*(1–2), 65–73.

Polit, D. F., Beck, C. T., & Hungler, B. P. (2001). *Essentials of nursing research: Methods, appraisal, and utilization (5th ed.)*. New York, NY: Lippincott.

Tolman, E. C. (1938). The determiners of behavior at a choice point. *Psychological Review, 45*(1), 1–41.

Toussaint, L., Barry, M., Bornfriend, L., & Markman, M. (2014). Restore: The journey toward self-forgiveness: A randomized trial of patient education on self-forgiveness in cancer patients and caregivers. *Journal of Health Care Chaplaincy, 20*(2), 54–74.

Vogt, W. P. (1993). *Dictionary of statistics and methodology: A nontechnical guide for the social sciences*. Thousand Oaks, CA: Sage Publications.

Measures of Central Tendency in Chaplaincy, Health Care, and Related Research

KATHERINE R. B. JANKOWSKIandKEVINJ.FLANNELLY

The three measures of central tendency are discussed in this article: the mode, the median, and the mean. These measures of central tendency describe data in different and important ways, in relation to the level of measurement (nominal, ordinal, interval, or ratio) used to obtain the data. The results of published research studies, thought experiments, and graphs of frequency and percentage distributions of data are used as examples to demonstrate and explain the similarities and differences among these summary measures of data. The examples include the application of nominal, ordinal, interval, and ratios scales to measure pain, anxiety, chaplaincy services, religious behaviors, and treatment-related preferences, and their respective measures of central tendency. Examples of unimodal and bimodal distributions, and differences in the relative locations of the median and mean in symmetrical and skewed distributions are also presented and discussed.

People who are ill have needs that vary from person to person, and it is important to identify these individual needs to provide the best evidence-based care. People who are ill may also have illness experiences and needs

TABLE 1 Measures of Central Tendency that can be Used With Different Levels of Measurement

Levels of Measurement	Measures of Central Tendency
Nominal Scales	Mode
Ordinal Scales	Mode, Median
Interval Scales	Mode, Median, Mean
Ratio Scales	Mode, Median, Mean

that are common for people within the context of their particular illness. For example, patients with stage IV cancer will have different needs in common with each other that are common with patients with heart disease. Surveys and interviews are often used to discover the needs of groups of people, and they are useful for obtaining information about the frequency of specific needs for people with specific illnesses. These needs can be assessed, for example, by the number of times cancer patients mention pain-related needs or the number of times heart disease patients mention life-style change needs. The needs mentioned most often by patients can be said to be the commonly expected needs of the groups.

Measures of central tendency provide measures of the common charac-teristics of groups. There are three measures of central tendency, the mode, the median, and the mean, each of which are unique and will be discussed, in turn. Only certain measures of central tendency can be used with different levels of measurement, as shown in Table 1.

THE MODE

The mode indicates the most frequently occurring object in a dataset or score on a variable, such as a response to a survey question. The mode is the only measure of central tendency that can accurately describe data on a nominal level of measurement. For example, a Pew survey (Pew, 2012) placed people into one of two categories, or groups: religiously "affiliated" or "unaffiliated," depending on whether they said "Yes" or "No" in response to the question: "Do you have a religious affiliation?" When each person, based on their answer to this one question, is put into one of these mutually exclusive nom-inal categories (affiliated or unaffiliated) the mode is the category that has the largest number of people. In the Pew (2012) survey results roughly 80% of the people said they were religiously affiliated and 20% said they were not affiliated. So, being affiliated with a religion was the modal response—the most frequent response—for those people surveyed by Pew.

Of course, people can be grouped in many ways using nominal scales— by their gender, their ethnicity, their profession, etc. (see the discussion of nominal scales in Flannelly, Flannelly, & Jankowski, 2014). Nominal scales are widely used in healthcare to classify diseases, treatments, and causes of death. It is possible to have ties for the most frequent nominal data category and, as such, there can be more than one mode in a data set. For example, when the Pew study asked religiously unaffiliated individuals about their political ideology, 38% said they were moderates and another 38% said they were liberals, thus the distribution was bimodal. The other survey respondents said they were conservatives or professed no political ideology. In another example, the Centers for Disease Control (Heron, 2013) reported that the leading cause of death in the United States in 2010 was heart disease (24%), which was just ahead of cancer (23%). Thus, the distribution of causes of death in the United States comes close to being a bimodal distribution, but technically there is only one mode (heart disease).

Nominal scales have been used to examine various aspects of healthcare, including patients' treatment preferences. An interesting example is a small study of prostate cancer patients (Mazur & Hickam, 1996). The researchers presented the patients with three mutually exclusive treatment-decision options, of which 53% of patients preferred surgery, 42% preferred symptom management, and 4% preferred to let their physician decide what treatment was best. This makes the surgery option the modal response. Another study of patient preferences compared the preferences of three groups of patients who were classified as being religious, non-religious, and "in between" (Ehman, Ott, Short, Ciampa, & Hansen-Flashen, 1999). The patients were asked if they wanted their doctor to talk to them about their spiritual or religious beliefs if they were gravely ill; the responses were grouped into three categories: agree, disagree, and undecided. The mode of the religious patients was agree (89%), the mode of the in-between patients was agree (63%), and the mode of non-religious patients was agree (50%), although the modes themselves were quite different.

To reiterate, the mode is the most frequent answer to a question, or class of objects/things (e.g., causes of death). It is the measure of central tendency that is used for nominal information, and it only provides information about the most frequent responses, categories, or classes of things. A unique property of the mode is that it is possible to have two modes in a distribution (called a bimodal distribution), whereas a distribution can have only one median and one mean.

THE MEDIAN

Many types of research questions require more than a simple "yes" or "no" answer. To achieve a finer level of understanding and analysis, researchers often ask people to rank their preference for something. A rank is a measure on the ordinal scale of measurement. For example, one might ask people to rank how they prefer their coffee from most to least preferred: black, black with sugar, with milk, with milk and sugar, or some other way (Varela, Beltrán, & Fiszman, 2014). A summary can then be made of the most preferred way to drink coffee for that group of people. Or one might ask people to rank their preference for different types of health education programs (Bech, Sørensen, & Lauridsen, 2005), so that the most preferred type of education program can be identified. Although the things being ranked in these two examples are quite different from one another, what is of interest is to identify the most preferred thing. Once the things are ranked, the ranks themselves can be used to identify the things of most importance, intermediate importance, and least importance among the things being ranked by a group.

A 2003 study of cancer patients asked the patients to rank the things that were most important to them when they were making a medical decision on how to best treat—with either chemotherapy or supportive care—their metastatic lung cancer. Their oncologist was asked to do the same (Silvestri, Knittig, Zoller, & Nietert, 2003). Table 2 shows the patients' and oncologists' rankings of the importance of seven factors they consider when choosing between the two potential treatments. The most important factor, the Cancer Doctor's Recommendation, was the most important factor for both patients and doctors, receiving an average rank of 1. Interestingly, Faith in God was the second most important factor for patients, but the least important factor for oncologists.

Side Effects was the median rank of patients, the absolute middle rank, since it was ranked fourth out of the seven factors. The factor that received the median rank for oncologists was Spouse's Input, since it was ranked fourth by them. The median rank is found by lining up the ranks of the things being evaluated in order of magnitude. In Table 2, the seven factors and their ranks are lined up in order of their ranks for the patients. It is possible to arrange the ranks from low to high (or high to low) because each rank reflects an increasing amount of some dimension, such as liking, preference or, in this instance, importance. However, the amount, or magnitude, of the difference between the scores is unspecified when things are ranked and, in practice, the ordinal level of measurement (i.e., rank ordering of preferences, importance, etc.) is used relatively rarely in healthcare research because the magnitude of the difference between the ranks is unspecified (see Flannelly

TABLE 2 Rankings of the Importance of Seven Factors When Choosing Between Two Potential Treatments

Ranking of Importance	Patient's Rank	Oncologist's Rank
Cancer Doctor's Recommendation	1	1
Faith in God	2	7
Ability to Cure	3	2
Side Effects	4	3
Family Doctor's Recommendation	5	5
Spouse's Input	6	4
Children's Input	7	6

et al., 2014). This characteristic of rankings severely restricts the types of statistical analyses that can be performed on ordinal scales, which restricts their use in research.

Another way to understand what people prefer, or how important something is to them, is to have them assign numbers to their responses to questions or statements. For example, in a study of religion and psychological well-being (Fry, 2000) people were asked to answer the question "How important is religion to you in your daily life?" by responding with a number between 1 and 6, in which 1 meant religion is not at all important and 6 meant religion is very important. Such questions are often rephrased to make statements (e.g., "Religion is important in my daily life.") and people can be asked how strongly they agree or disagree with the statements (e.g., 1 = strongly disagree, 2 = disagree, 3 = agree, and 4 = strongly agree). Subjective measures of health have used a similar technique. For instance, one of the questions on the SF-36 [see the explanation of the SF-36 given by Flannelly et al. (2014)] states "I am as healthy as anyone I know," to which respondents are asked to rate their level of agreement or disagreement. These kinds of rating scales are usually treated as interval scales because the assigned values are assumed to reflect subjectively equal intervals. The study by Fry is particularly valuable as an example because it used similar scales to measure other aspects of religion, including how often study participants attended religious services (from 1 = never to 6 = daily), and how involved participants were with their church or synagogue (from 1 = marginally involved to 6 = deeply involved).

We will use a thought experiment to give an example of a median, and compare the median to the mode. Let's imagine a rating scale in which patients indicate the amount of pain they are currently feeling. The scale would use pictures of faces to represent different levels of pain, from feeling no pain to feeling excruciating pain; some examples of this type of pain rating scale use faces, such as those used in studies by da Silva, Thuler, and de Leon-Casasola (2011) and Wilson and Helgadottir (2006). Both of these articles used a pain rating scale that had six faces. However, to demonstrate the properties of the median and mode more easily we will imagine a pain rating scale with eleven faces. At one end of this scale "no pain" is represented by a pleasant or happy face with the number 0 below the face, the exact middle point of the scale has a face that is impassive, with no emotion and the number 5 below this face, and the other end of the scale has a picture of a very upset, agonized face with the number 10 below this face. The subjective judgment of zero pain on the scale is assumed to indicate the complete absence of pain: see discussion by Flannelly et al. (2014) about zero points in interval and ratio scales.

On such a 0–10 scale, the exact middle point of the scale is the number 5, as there are five smaller numbers to the left of the 5, and five higher numbers to the right of the 5. Eleven people could each select one of the 11 numbers

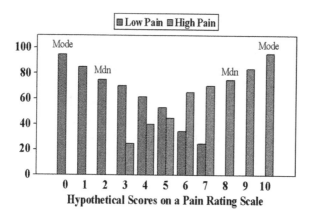

FIGURE 1 Frequency distributions of the hypothetical scores of high and low pain groups on a pain rating scale.

from 0 to 10 and the median of this group would be 5. If 22 people selected pain ratings, and two people selected 0, two people selected 1, two selected 2, and so on through the values 0–10, the median of this group's data would still be 5. This is due to the fact that since the number of respondents is an even number (i.e., 22), and everyone chose one of the 11 pain ratings, the median is the value at middle of the scale.

We can take our thought experiment further by pretending we have two groups of persons who complete the pain scale: those with "Low Pain" and those with "High Pain." Figure 1 plots the frequency distribution of the scores of these two pain groups, with each pain-group consisting of 500 persons. The majority of the scores of the low-pain group are primarily at the low end of the scale, and no one has a score higher than 7. By lining up the scores in order one finds that the median score (or middle score) of the low-pain group is 2 (Mdn). For the high-pain group, the majority of the scores are primarily at the high end of the scale, and no one has a score lower than 3. By lining up the scores in order one finds that the median score of the high-pain group is 8 (Mdn). Figure 1 also shows the modes for the two groups. Zero was the most frequent pain rating for the low-pain group, with just over 90 people rating their pain as 0, so zero is the mode for the low-pain group. In the high-pain group the most frequent pain rating was 10, with over 90 people rating their pain as 10, so 10 is the mode for the high-pain group.

The two distributions are said to be skewed because they are not symmetrical. The scores of the low-pain group trail-off toward the higher values of the scale, and, therefore, the distribution is said to be positively skewed. The scores of the high-pain group trail-off toward the lower values of the scale, and, therefore, the distribution is said to be negatively skewed.

To summarize, the median is the mid-point of a series of data points arranged in order of magnitude from low to high (or high to low). The median is the mid-point of any distribution of scores, with 50% of the scores falling below the median and 50% falling above the median. As it is simply the absolute middle value in a distribution, the median is not affected by the shape of the distribution or by extremely large or extremely small scores in the distribution. Because the median is the exact mid-point of a distribution it is commonly used in health research to divide distributions in half, usually referred to as a median-split, for certain types statistical analyses. The median can be used as a measure of central tendency for ordinal, interval, and ratio data.

THE MEAN

The mean is the most widely used measure of central tendency. It can be used with both interval and ratio levels of measurement. Quite simply, the mean is the arithmetic average: the sum of the scores divided by the number of scores. It takes into account all the information available in the data; the number of observations and the value of each observation. In doing so the mean provides a different kind of measure of the center of a distribution of scores, which gives it a privileged place in research. It is very useful for many types of statistical analyses, including comparisons of groups at one or more points in time.

The mean complements the mode and median. Whenever there are large differences between the values of the mean, the median, and the mode, researchers are informed that the data are complex and require careful interpretation. An example of how the mean provides different information from the median can be seen in the results of a study of chaplaincy visits in acute and non-acute hospital settings (Handzo et al., 2008). This study collected data from more than 34,000 chaplain visits in 13 hospitals over the course of 3 years. The number of minutes was recorded for each chaplain's visit with patients when the patient was alone, with family, or with family and friends.

The study found that the median and mean duration (number of minutes) of chaplains' visits in both the acute and nonacute settings were different, and that the means were larger. This indicates that some chaplain visits were substantially longer than the medians indicate. The substantially greater time of some chaplaincy visits increased the mean relative to the median. Specifically, as can be seen in Table 4 of the study of Handzo et al. (2008), the median (Md) visit duration of chaplains' visits in acute hospital settings was 10 minutes regardless of whether the patient was alone, with family, or with family and friends. The mean number of minutes was higher than the median in all three circumstances (14.1, 15.0, and 15.5 minutes, respectively). In the nonacute healthcare setting, the medians (5, 5, and 10 minutes, respectively) and means (8.3, 10.3, and 9.9 minutes, respectively) were equal to or smaller than those in the acute care settings. The mean visit duration that was the shortest was when the patient was seen alone in the non-acute setting (8.3 minutes).

The differences between the medians and the means in the aforementioned example are due to the fact that the mathematical average takes into account the actual values of the data points—the number of minutes in a chaplain's visit, whereas the median only looks at the data point in the exact middle of an ordered line-up of the data (the number of minutes in each visit ordered from low to high). The actual number of minutes of a visit by a chaplain varies greatly in this data as can be seen in a second article published on these data (Vanderwerker, Handzo, Fogg, & Overvold, 2009). The left side of Table 6 of Vanderwerker et al. shows the distribution of chaplain visit durations in acute healthcare settings. As seen in Table 6, chaplain visits ranged in duration from 5 minutes to 2 hours.

Because different measures of central tendency provide different kinds of information about data distributions, one has to decide on the best measure of central tendency when measuring healthcare variables (such chaplain visits) from a clinical and/or administrative perspective. To bring our discussion of the differences between modes, medians and means home, Figure 2 presents hypothetical data to demonstrate how the mean, median, and mode might differ in a given distribution of scores. The example illustrates hypothetical distributions of anxiety in the general population and in hospitalized patients, using a hypothetical 0–10 scale like the pain scale used in our earlier example. Many studies have examined anxiety in the general population and in hospitalized patients in the United States (see literature reviewed in Gaudette & Jankowski, 2013).

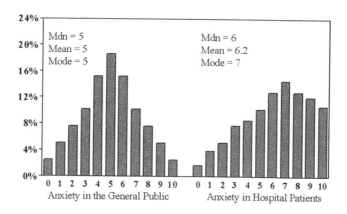

FIGURE 2 Percentage distributions of hypothetical anxiety scores among the general public and hospitalized patients.

The left side of Figure 2 depicts the hypothetical distribution of anxiety scores in the U.S. general public on a 0–10 scale. As is the case with pain rating scales, the subjective judgment of zero anxiety on this hypothetical scale is assumed to indicate the complete absence of pain: see discussion by Flannelly et al. (2014) regarding zero points in interval and ratio scales.

Figure 2 shows that the distribution of anxiety in the general public is relatively symmetrical about the mean. Given that this distribution is symmetrically distributed about the mean, the mean, median and mode are all located at the middle of the distribution; in this case, they are all represented by a score of 5. Anxiety has been found to be very common among hospital patients (see Gaudette & Jankowski, 2013), and it tends to be higher than in the general public. This higher anxiety of hospital patients is reflected in the hypothetical illustration of the distribution of anxiety scores in right side of Figure 2. The hypothetical distributions were created to illustrate differences that can be found between the mean, median, and mode in distributions with different shapes. Hence, the distribution of patient anxiety was created so that the mode of patient anxiety is 7, the median is 6, and the mean lies in between the median and mode. The Figure also shows that the median is one point higher, and the mode is two points higher in graph of patient anxiety scores than the graph of anxiety among the general public.

To reiterate, in a symmetrical distribution of data, such as can be seen in the left bar graph, the mean, median and mode are likely to be the same. However, there often is a discrepancy between the location of the mode, median, and the mathematical average (i.e., mean), as is depicted in the right bar graph. As in the example of the high pain group in Figure 1, the anxiety scores of patients in Figure 2 are negatively skewed. Figure 1 of a *JHCC* article by Spidell et al. (2011) shows the actual findings of a study on grief among chaplains, in which the results are positively skewed. That figure plots the distribution of negative coping scores (i.e., number of negative coping behaviors) found in the study. The number of possible coping behaviors range from 0 to 12, with a median and mode of 3. Our best estimate of the mean number of negative behaviors, based on the graph, is 3.6.

To summarize, the mean is the arithmetic average of data that are in the form of numbers measured on interval or ratio scales. The mean takes into account the values of the numbers to arrive at a measure that represents the middle, or center, of the distribution of data. It is different from the mode, which is the most frequently occurring score or other form of data, and the median, which is the absolute center of all the data ordered from low to high or high to low.

SUMMARY AND CONCLUSION

Each measure of central tendency is an important measure of a dataset and provides valuable information about the variables that are represented in the dataset. The most common symptom, the average chaplaincy visit, the most frequent length of chaplains' visits, and a patient's preferred treatment regimen can all be identified using measures of central tendency. Thankfully, researchers have computers with statistical programs to calculate the mode, median, and mean of any number of variables, such as measures of pain, anxiety, or duration of visits, for any number of people. The computer arranges the values in order and by their frequency to quickly provide us with the most frequent value (the mode), the value that divides the distribution of scores in half (the median), and calculates the average value of all the scores (the mean). Computers are especially helpful with large datasets, such as those analyzed by Handzo et al. (2008) and Vanderwerker et al. (2009).

With measures of central tendency we can record and measure and make meaning out of information at a group level; we can describe and compare groups. With more advanced statistics we can introduce control into our comparisons and refine our conclusions. We can predict outcomes based on what we know about many different variables. However, statistics are only as useful as the appropriateness of their application to data. We must be careful to use the mode, median, and mean appropriately. Computer programs, for example, will calculate the mean of nominal data even though it does not make sense to do so; hence, it is up to the researcher to know when a mean is appropriate and when the mode or median is the most appropriate measure of central tendency. It is hoped that this article has provided a basic understanding of how these central tendency statistics are derived and used, and, as a result, facilitates the proper use of the measures of central tendency.

REFERENCES

Bech, M., Sørensen, J., & Lauridsen, J. (2005). Eliciting women's preferences for a training program in breast self-examination: A conjoint ranking experiment. *Value in Health*, 8(4), 479–487. doi:10.1111/j.1524–4733.2005.00039.x

da Silva, F. C., Thuler, L. C. S., & de Leon-Casasola, O. A. (2011). Validity and reliability of two pain assessment tools in Brazilian children and adolescents. *Journal of Clinical Nursing*, 20, 1842–1848. doi:10.1111/j.1365–2702. 2010.03662.x

Ehman, J. W., Ott, B. B., Short, T. H., Ciampa, R. C., & Hansen-Flaschen, J. (1999). Do patients want physicians to inquire about their spiritual or religious beliefs if they become gravely ill? *Archives of Internal Medicine*, 159(15), 1803–1806. doi:10.1001/archinte.159.15.1803

Flannelly, L. T., Flannelly, K. J., & Jankowski, K. R. B. (2014). Fundamentals of measurement in healthcare research. *Journal of Health Care Chaplaincy*, 20(2), 75–82.

Fry, P. S. (2000). Religious involvement, spirituality and personal meaning for life: Existential predictors of psychological wellbeing in community-residing and institutional care elders. *Aging & Mental Health*, 4(4), 375–387. doi:10.1080/713649965

Gaudette, H., & Jankowski, K. R. B. (2013). Spiritual coping and anxiety in palliative care patients: A pilot study. *Journal of Health Care Chaplaincy, 19*(4), 131–139. doi:10.1080/08854726.2013.823785

Handzo, G. F., Flannelly, K. J., Murphy, K. M., Bauman, J. P., Oettinger, S. M., Goodell, S. E., … Jacobs, M. R. (2008). What do chaplains really do? I. Visitation in the New York chaplaincy study. *Journal of Health Care Chaplaincy, 14*(1), 20–38. doi:10.1080/08854720802053838

Heron, M. (2013). Deaths: Leading causes for 2010. *National Vital Statistics Reports 62*(6). Retrieved from the World Wide Web at http://www.cdc.gov/nchs/data/nvsr/nvsr62/nvsr62_06.pdf November 11, 2014.

Mazur, D. J., & Hickam, D. H. (1996). Patient preferences for management of localized prostate cancer. *Western Journal of Medicine, 165*(1–2), 26–30.

Pew. (2012). *"Nones" on the rise: One-in-five adults have no religious affiliation.* Retrieved from the World Wide Web at http://www.pewforum.org/files/2012/10/NonesOnTheRise-full.pdf July 15, 2014.

Silvestri, G. A., Knittig, S., Zoller, J. S., & Nietert, P. J. (2003). Importance of faith on medical decisions regarding cancer care. *Journal of Clinical Oncology, 21*(7), 1379–1382. doi:10.1200/jco.2003.08.036

Spidell, S., Wallace, A., Carmack, C. L., Nogueras-González, G. M., Parker, C. L., & Cantor, S. B. (2011). Grief in healthcare chaplains: An investigation of the presence of disenfranchised grief. *Journal of Health Care Chaplaincy, 17*(1–2), 75–86. doi:10.1080/08854726.2011.559859

Vanderwerker, L. C., Handzo, G. F., Fogg, S. L., & Overvold, J. A. (2009). Selected findings from the "New York" and the "Metropolitan" chaplaincy studies: A 10-year comparison of chaplaincy in the New York City area. *Journal of Health Care Chaplaincy, 15*(1), 13–24. doi:10.1080/08854720802698483

Varela, P., Beltrán, J., & Fiszman, S. (2014). An alternative way to uncover drivers of coffee liking: Preference mapping based on consumers' preference ranking and open comments. *Food Quality and Preference, 32*, 152–159. doi:10.1016/j.foodqual.2013.03.004

Wilson, M. E., & Helgadóttir, H. L. (2006). Patterns of pain and analgesic use in 3- to 7-year-old children after tonsillectomy. *Pain Management Nursing, 7*(4), 159–166. doi:10.1016/j.pmn.2006.09.005

Measures of Variability in Chaplaincy, Health Care, and Related Research

KEVIN J. FLANNELLY, KATHERINE R. B. JANKOWSKI
and LAURA T. FLANNELLY

This article discusses statistical measures of variability in relation to measures of central tendency and levels of measurement. Three measures of variability used in healthcare research (the range, the interquartile range, and the standard deviation) are described and compared, including their uses and limitations. The article describes how each of the three measures is calculated, and it provides a step-by-step example of calculating the sums of squares, variance, and standard deviation. Graphs of frequency and percentage distributions are used to show how the interquartile range and the standard deviation represent the variability observed within distributions. The article discusses the properties of the normal curve regarding the distribution of scores around the mean in relation to the standard deviation, and illustrates differences in the shapes of normal curves with the same mean but different standard deviations.

An earlier article in the Research Methodology section of *JHCC* explained measures of central of tendency (Jankowski & Flannelly, 2015). Measures of central tendency are statistics that use a single number to summarize a

---

Color versions of one or more of the figures in the article can be found online at www.tandfonline.com/whcc.

distribution of scores, or values, on some variable. As that article explained, only certain measures of central tendency may be used to describe variables using different levels of measurement. Nominal data can only be summarized by their mode; ordinal data may be summarized by their mode and median; and interval and ratio data may be summarized by their mode, median, and mean.

The current article complements that article by explaining how a researcher summarizes the variability (also known as dispersion, or spread) of a distribution of scores on a variable. We will start by using examples based on the hypothetical pain scale described in that article. The scale measures subjective pain by asking patients to rate the level of pain they are currently experiencing from 0 to 10. For expository purposes, we assume that the difference between each value on the scale (the ratings of pain) are equal intervals; for example, that the difference in pain between a rating of 1 and a rating of 2 is equal to the difference in pain between a rating of 8 and a rating of 9. We further assume that the value 0 is the complete absence of pain, such that a rating of 4 is twice as much pain as a rating of 2, and a rating of 8 is twice as much pain as a rating of 4. The first assumption is that the scale represents at least an interval level of measurement, and the second assumption is that the scale specifically represents a ratio level of measurement. The hypothetical scale is comparable to scales that are actually used with patients to measure pain (e.g., da Silva, Thuler, & de Leon-Casasola, 2011; Wilson & Helgadóttir, 2006), although the clinicians and researchers who use them may or may not make these two assumptions.

Imagine that 10 patients who completed a pain scale reported the levels of pain shown in the left column (Sample 1). Imagine that a second sample of patients reported the pain scores shown in the right column (Sample 2). Obviously, the two distributions of pain scores are very different (see Table 1). The scores of Sample 1 are spread across all values of the scale (0–10), whereas the scores of Sample 2 are all at the midpoint of the scale.

TABLE 1 Mean hypothetical pain ratings of two samples

	Sample 1	Sample 2	
	0	5	
	1	5	
	2	5	
	3	5	
	4	5	
	5	5	
	6	5	
	7	5	
	8	5	
	9	5	
	10	5	
Σ =	55	55	(sum of the scores)
N =	11	11	(number of scores)
Σ/N =	5	5	(mean of the scores)

Although the shapes of the two distributions are very different, if we calculate the means, or averages of the two samples, the means are identical; the mean of each sample is 5. The median (i.e., the middle score of the series of scores) of the two distributions also is 5. Thus, we see that the mean and median do not provide information about the variation among the scores in the distributions. Hence, just knowing the mean or median of a distribution is not enough information to understand the nature of the distribution.

Measures of variability provide information about the distribution of scores of a variable that is not provided by measures of central tendency. The *range* is the simplest measure of variability and it can be used with ordinal, interval, and ratio scales; there is no measure of variability for nominal scales (Sharma, 2005; Spence, Cotton, Underwood, & Duncan, 1990). The *range* is the difference between the highest and lowest scores, although studies often use the term "range" when they display the lowest and highest scores (e.g., range $= 0$–10), instead of showing the difference between them (e.g., range $= 10$).

As the *range* is the difference between the highest and lowest scores, it would be useful to know the *range* in instances like the distributions in Table 1, if we could not see the actual distributions of the scores. As the *range* of Sample 1 is 10 and the *range* of Sample 2 is 0, the *range* tells us that the patients in Sample 1 reported the full range of the possible pain scores on the scale, whereas all of the patients in Sample 2 reported the identical score. However, knowing the *range* is not always as useful as it was here. The *range*, for example, does not permit us to tell the difference between the two distributions shown in Figure 1.

Figure 1 shows the hypothetical distributions of pain ratings from two different samples of patients. Each distribution contains 150 ratings between

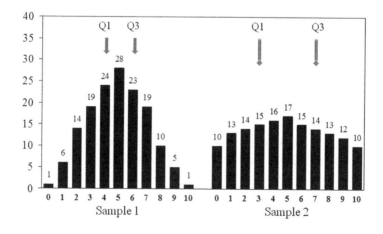

FIGURE 1 Hypothetical frequency distributions of pain ratings from two samples of patients.

and 0 and 10; the distributions were created to be roughly symmetrical with a mean, median, and mode = 5. However, their shapes are quite different. The ratings in Sample 1 are clustered around the mean rating of 5, and the frequency (or number) of ratings fall-off rapidly, moving away from the mean. The frequencies of the ratings in Sample 2, on the other hand, are much more evenly distributed across the eleven possible ratings. Nevertheless, as the *range* is the difference between the lowest and highest ratings in this distribution, the *range* of both distributions is 10. Hence, the range does not let us know that the shapes of the distributions are different.

Another measure of variability may be more helpful: the *interquartile range (IQR)* (Dawson-Saunders & Trapp, 1994; Sharma, 2005). Though the name may seem very technical, the concept is actually quite simple. To find the IQR, the first step is to divide the distribution into four groups of ratings. Starting from the lowest rating, each quartile contains a 25% portion of the total number of ratings. The scores at the exact points of 25, 50, 75, and 100% of any distribution of scores are known as the quartiles. Therefore, the second step is to find the units of measurement of the 0–10 ratings in our example that contain the middle 50% of the ratings: that is, those falling within the first (Q1) and third (Q3) quartiles. As each distribution in Figure 1 consists of 150 ratings, we want to know where the middle half of the ratings are located, in this case where the 75 ratings around the middle are located. As the distributions were specially created for this article to make the medians (the middle score of a distribution) the same in each distribution, we can start from the middle rating and count the number of ratings on either side of the median.

In Sample 1, 28 patients had the median score of 5, 24 had a score of 4, and 23 had a score of 6 (28 + 24 + 23 = 75). The middle 50% of ratings are between 4 and 6. The final step is to calculate the *interquartile range*: IQR = Q3 − Q1; as Q3 is 6 and Q1 = 4, the *interquartile range* = 2. That is, 50% of the rating scores fall within two values of the median. In Sample 2, 15 patients had a rating of 3, 16 had a rating of 4, 17 had the median rating of 5, 15 had a rating of 6, and 14 had a rating of 7. As a result, half of the ratings of Sample 2 in Figure 1 are between 4 and 7 (15 + 16 + 17 + 15 + 14 = 77). A rating of 4 is the upper boundary of Q1 and a rating of 7 is the upper boundary of Q3, therefore, the *interquartile range* for Sample 2 is 7−3 = 4. Hence, the *IQR* shows that the spread of the ratings is larger in Sample 2 (*IQR* = 4) than Sample 1 (*IQR* = 2). Researchers sometimes report the *semi-interquartile range*, which simply means that they divided the *interquartile range* by 2 (Sharma, 2005; Spence et al., 1990).

The *IQR* is useful because it provides a relative measure of differences in the variability of distributions, and it can be applied to ordinal, interval, and ratio scales. However, it ignores scores outside the first and third quarters of the distribution, therefore, it is not suited for statistically comparing differences in the distributions of samples.

It would be useful to have a measure of variability that captures the variation among all the scores in a distribution. One way to show the variation in the scores of a distribution that are measured on interval or ratio scales might be to show how the scores vary from their mean (deviation scores). This might be done, as shown in Table 2.

The first step would be to calculate the mean (M) of the scores (X's), which are shown in the first column on the left. The sum (Σ) of the scores equals 21, and the number (N) of scores equals 7, and, therefore, the mean (M) equals 3. If we place the mean in the second column (M) we can subtract the mean from each score ($X - M$) to calculate the distance of each score from the mean (the deviations scores), which might give us a measure of the variation of the scores around the mean, by summing the differences from the mean and taking their average. In case you did not see the zero mean coming, it can be explained by the fact that deviation scores above and below the mean cancel each other out, so they sum to zero, and consequently, their mean equals zero.

However, if we ignored the signs of the differences, and used the absolute value of the deviations scores we would obtain a statistic that reflects the variation of scores about the mean that does not cancel itself out (Sharma, 2005), as seen in Table 3. Following the steps shown in Table 2, we calculate the mean and then subtract it from each score to obtain the deviation scores ($X - M$). The next step ignores the signs of the deviation scores to obtain the absolute difference ($|X - M|$) between each score and the mean. This allows us to calculate the mean of the absolute deviation scores, which, in this example is about 1.7.

This approach would seem to be good way to avoid the problem that the mean of the actual deviations scores is always equal to zero. However, taking the absolute values of the deviation scores is the mathematical equivalent of multiplying the scores below the mean by -1, such that a portion of the scores are transformed and another portion of scores are not transformed. This makes it impossible to use this statistic, called the mean deviation or average deviation, in further calculations (Sharma, 2005; Spence et al., 1990).

TABLE 2 Mean of each score's deviation from the mean

	X	M	X – M
	0	3	−3
	1	3	−2
	2	3	−1
	3	3	0
	4	3	+1
	5	3	+2
	6	3	+3
$\Sigma =$	21		0
$N =$	7		7
$\Sigma/N =$	3		0

TABLE 3 Mean of the absolute deviation scores

	X	M	X − M	|X − M|
	0	3	−3	3
	1	3	−2	2
	2	3	−1	1
	3	3	0	0
	4	3	+1	1
	5	3	+2	2
	6	3	+3	3
Σ =	21			12
N =	7			7
Σ/N =	3			1.7

The most commonly used statistic to express the variability of scores measured on interval or ratio scales is the *standard deviation*. The calculation of the *standard deviation* entails making the deviation scores positive by squaring each one so that their mean can be calculated. The procedures for calculating the *standard deviation* are shown in Table 4.

The initial steps are the same as those shown in Tables 2 and 3. The mean is calculated and subtracted from each score ($X − M$). The next step is to square the deviation scores to make them all positive numbers: $(X − M)^2$. The sum of the squared deviations from the mean is called the *sum of squares* (or *SS*), which is used in a variety of statistical analyses and tests. The mean of the squared deviations is called the *variance*, which is also used in a number of statistical procedures. The *standard deviation* is the square root of the *variance*, which puts the *standard deviation* back into the same units as the mean.

We did not mention earlier that the distributions of the samples in Figure 1 were also designed to have different *standard deviations* (SD). Sample 1 has an SD of 2 and Sample 2 has an SD of 3. Although the samples have the same means (5), medians (5), modes (5), and ranges (10), the

TABLE 4 Calculating the standard deviation of the scores

	X	M	X − M	$(X − M)^2$	
	0	3	−3	9	
	1	3	−2	4	
	2	3	−1	1	
	3	3	0	0	
	4	3	+1	1	
	5	3	+2	4	
	6	3	+3	9	
Σ =	21			28	(sum of squares)
N =	7			7	
Σ/N =	3			4	(variance)
√Σ/N =				2	(standard deviation)

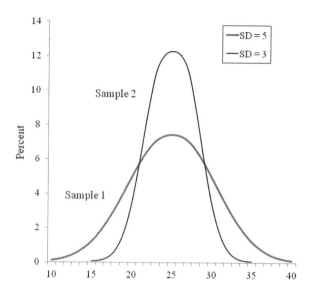

FIGURE 2 Percentage distributions (normal curves) with different standard deviations.

different shapes of the distributions account for their different SDs. The SDs of the distributions may also differ because the samples contain different range of scores, even if they have the same mean, median, and mode, and the same basic shape.

The distributions of the samples in Figure 2 purposely were created to illustrate distributions with the same means, medians, and modes, but different ranges and SDs. The distributions are close approximations to what is called a *normal curve,* or *Gaussian distribution,* in which the shape of the curve and the proportion of the area under different portions of the curve (and therefore, the percentage of scores) are directly related to the SD of the distribution.

Figure 2 contains two hypothetical distributions of scores from samples of the general public who completed an anxiety scale that has a minimum score of 10 and a maximum score of 40. As can be seen in the figure, Sample 1 encompasses all possible scores on the scale, and, therefore, the range of the distribution is 30, as the *range* is the value of the highest score minus the value of the lowest score. The distribution of the scores of Sample 1 was created to have a SD of 5 and to be the shape of a *normal curve.* A unique property of the *normal curve* (or *normal distribution*) is that 99.7% of the scores of the distribution fall within three SDs of either side of the mean, and 95,5% of the scores of fall within two SDs of either side of the mean. Over two-thirds of the scores (68.2%) fall within one SD of the mean of a normal curve (Alder & Roessler, 1968). As the distribution of Sample 1 includes all the possible scores (i.e., 10–40) on the anxiety scale, 100% of the scores in the sample fall within three SDs of the sample's mean.

As the mean of Sample 1 is a score of 25, one SD below the mean is a score of 20 and one SD above the mean is a score of 30. Therefore, 68.2% of the scores in Sample 1 fall between 20 and 30. Similarly, as two SDs below the mean is a score of 15 and two SDs above the mean is a score of 35, 95.5% of the scores in Sample 1 fall between 15 and 35.

Sample 2 has a mean of 25, a standard deviation of 3, and a mean of 25, and, therefore, one SD below the mean is a score of 22 and one standard deviation above the mean is a score of 28. Hence, 68.2% of the scores in Sample 2 fall between 22 and 28. Similarly, as two SDs below the mean is a score of 19 and two SDs above the mean is a score of 31, 95.5% of the scores fall between 19 and 31.

The differences in the shapes of the two distributions in Figure 2 illustrate that the shape of a normal curve differs depending on its SD. Distributions with larger SDs are relatively flat, or *platykurtic*, whereas distributions with smaller SDs are relatively steep, or *leptokurtic*. Of course, not all distributions are symmetrical (see Jankowski & Flannelly, 2015), or normally distributed. This is an important point because differences in the shapes and SDs of distributions affect what type of statistical analyses a researcher should choose to compare the scores of different samples.

CONCLUSIONS

Measures of variability regarding the mean are critical statistics for understanding distributions of scores (i.e., data). The *range, interquartile range, standard deviation,* and the *normal curve* allow researchers to know how many scores are near the middle of a distribution, how many scores are away from the middle, and how far out from the middle the scores might land.

In essence, measures of variability provide numerical pictures of the data that describe the spread of the data about the mean. Measures of central tendency (the mean, median, and mode) are important statistics that provide a starting point for picturing the data, whereas measures of variability complete the numerical painting of the data.

In addition to the numerical description provided by measures of variability, the measure of variability called the *standard deviation* provides researchers an important statistic that can be used to compare two or more samples of scores using different types of statistical analyses. The selection of the types of statistical analyses that should be used to compare samples depends, in part, on their standard deviations and the shapes of their distributions.

REFERENCES

Alder, H. L., & Roessler, E. B. (1968). *Introduction to probability and statistics* (4th ed.). San Francisco, CA: W.H. Freeman.

Dawson-Saunders, B., & Trapp, R. G. (1994). *Basic and clinical biostatistics* (2nd ed.). Norwalk, CT: Appleton & Lange.

da Silva, F. C., Thuler, L. C. S., & de Leon-Casasola, O. A. (2011). Validity and reliability of two pain assessment tools in Brazilian children and adolescents. *Journal of Clinical Nursing*, 20, 1842–1848. doi:10.1111/j.1365–2702.2010.03662.x

Jankowski, K. R. B., & Flannelly, K. J. (2015). Measures of central tendency in chaplaincy, health care, and related research. *Journal of Health Care Chaplaincy*, 21 (1), 39–49. doi:10.1080/08854726.2014.989799

Sharma, A. K. (2005). *Text book of biostatistics I*. New Delhi, India: Discovery Publishing House.

Spence, J. T., Cotton, J. W., Underwood, B. J., & Duncan, C. P. (1990). *Elementary statistics* (5th ed.). Englewood Cliffs, NJ: Prentice-Hall.

Wilson, M. E., & Helgadóttir, H. L. (2006). Patterns of pain and analgesic use in 3- to 7-year-old children after tonsillectomy. *Pain Management Nursing*, 7 (4), 159–166. doi:10.1016/j. pmn.2006.09.005

Studying Associations in Health Care Research

KEVIN J. FLANNELLY, LAURA T. FLANNELLY
andKATHERINER.B.JANKOWSKI

This article discusses some of the types of relationships observed in healthcare research and depicts them in graphic form. The article begins by explaining two basic associations observed in chemistry and physics (Boyles' Law and Charles' Law), and illustrates how these associations are similar to curvilinear and linear associations, respectively, found in healthcare. Graphs of curvilinear associations include morbidity curves and survival and mortality curves. Several examples of linear relationships are given and methods of testing linear relationships with interval and ratio data are introduced (i.e., correlation and ordinary least-squares regression). In addition, 2×2 contingency tables for testing the association between categorical (or nominal) data are described. Finally, Sir Austin Bradford Hill's eight criteria for assessing causality from research on associations between variables are presented and explained. Three appendices provide interested readers with opportunities to practice interpreting selected curvilinear and linear relationships.

Color versions of one or more of the figures in the article can be found online at www.tandfonline.com/whcc.

INTRODUCTION

Most of science is devoted to trying to understand the relationships among things. You probably remember some of these scientific relationships from whatever science courses you took in high school or college. If you studied chemistry or physics, you might remember that the volume of a gas is related to temperature and pressure (Chakrabarty, 2001; Kumar, 2009). Thus, we will start with these scientific relationships as a way to introduce the study of associations between variables in healthcare research.

The Irish chemist Robert Boyle experimentally established the relationship between pressure and the volume of a gas in the early 1660s, and it has come to be known as Boyle's Law. However, the relationship between temperature and the volume of a gas was not established until 140 years later. The relationship between temperature and volume is called Charles's Law, after the French physicist Jacques Charles who conducted experiments in the 1780s. However, the relationship was not experimentally confirmed until 1802 by Joseph Gay-Lussac, another Frenchman (Cajori, 1917). These relationships have come to be called laws because they can be, and are defined by, mathematical formulas. Figures 1 and 2 are drawn to convey a general impression of the relationships, and not to provide an accurate representation of the underlying mathematical formulas.

Specifically, the volume of a gas is directly related to temperature, and inversely related to pressure. Thus, if you filled a balloon with a gas (such as oxygen or helium) in a room in which you could increase the temperature, the volume of the gas would increase if you kept the air pressure in the room constant.

This is illustrated in Figure 1, where the balloon becomes larger as the temperature in the room increases, holding the air pressure in the room constant. If, on the other hand, you kept the temperature of the room constant,

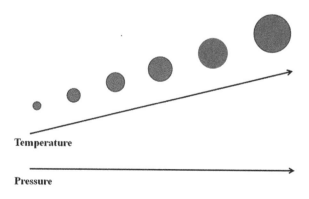

Temperature

Pressure

FIGURE 1 Increasing volume of a gas in a balloon with increasing ambient temperature, when the ambient pressure is constant.

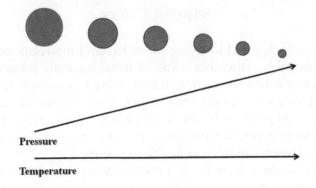

FIGURE 2 Decreasing volume of a gas in a balloon with increasing ambient pressure, when ambient temperature is constant.

and you increased the air pressure in the room, the balloon would get smaller, as generally illustrated in Figure 2.

These relationships between the volume of a gas and ambient temperature, and the volume of a gas and pressure are portrayed more accurately in Figure 3, using a standard graphic display. The numerical measurement of the volume of a gas (the dependent variable) is plotted on the ordinate (the vertical axis or y-axis) and the numerical measurements of temperature and pressure (the independent variables) are plotted on the abscissa (the horizontal axis or x-axis). Each line represents a series of specific points (not shown) that contains two bits of information in relation to each other: volume and temperature in A, and volume and pressure in B.

The overall relationship between volume and temperature in the graph is positive and linear (Charles's Law) on the Kelvin (°K) scale of temperature. The overall relationship between volume and pressure is a negative curvilinear relationship (Boyles' Law). Relationships between variables in health-care research may be curvilinear or linear relationships, and some are

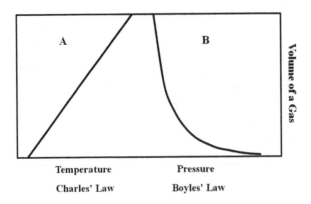

FIGURE 3 Relationship of the volume of a gas with temperature and pressure.

positive relationships, such as temperature and volume, whereas some are negative relationships, like volume and pressure. We will discuss curvilinear relationships in healthcare shortly, but here it is important to note that all three variables shown in Figure 3 (volume, temperature, and pressure) are continuous variables that are measured on ratio scales. As Flannelly, Flannelly, and Jankowski (2014a) discussed in a previous article on research methodology in the *Journal of Health Care Chaplaincy*, this means that the lowest point on each of the scales is a true zero (0 volume, 0 temperature, and 0 pressure) and that a one unit increase in each of the scales represents an equal interval increase in measurement.

TYPES OF ASSOCIATIONS IN HEALTHCARE RESEARCH

Relationships roughly similar to the convex curvilinear relationship between the volume of a gas and pressure are frequently observed in health research, particularly research on survival time. Survival time is a common measure of how long patients live after receiving a disease diagnosis; however, the slope of the curve is usually not as steep as the one shown in Figure 3 (Chen et al., 2013; Jordan, Fagliano, Rechtman, Lefkowitz, & Kaye, 2015). See Appendix 1 for further discussion and examples.

Figure 4 illustrates two other forms of curvilinear relationships that are often found in epidemiological research. The classic sigmoidal or S-shaped curve shown in Figure 4A is often seen when epidemiologists plot the cumulative number of cases diagnosed with a communicable disease over the time-course of the disease's outbreak (morbidity) (Gong et al., 2014; Guo et al., 2016). Cumulative mortality may also exhibit an S-shaped curve during the outbreak of a communicable disease, but cumulative mortality often tends to take the shape of the concave curvilinear relationship presented in Figure 4B. The curve in Figure 4B is particularly common when plotting

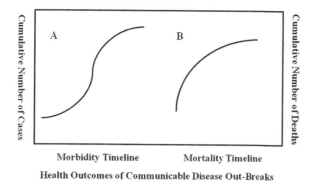

Health Outcomes of Communicable Disease Out-Breaks

FIGURE 4 Curvilinear relationships commonly observed in research on morbidity and mortality.

cumulative deaths from a life-threatening disease (Gammelager et al., 2012; Gibson & Robison, 2015). Mortality curves are basically the opposite of survival-time curves. See Appendix 2 for more discussion of these examples.

Most survey research in healthcare, as well as the social sciences, is designed to examine linear relationships between variables. This is typically done using two related types of statistical techniques, "regression" and "correlation" (Kleinbaum, Kupper, Muller, & Nuzam, 1998), which will be explained in greater detail in a later article. Simply put, linear regression, specifically, ordinary least-squares (OLS) regression, determines whether a linear relationship exists between two variables by: (a) plotting a straight line (a trend line) that best describes the association between the data on the two variables, and then (b) testing how close the data come to falling on the straight line. Correlation techniques, on the other hand, essentially assume the association between two variables is linear and tests the strength of the association between the two variables under this assumption (Kleinbaum et al., 1998). OLS regression and different correlation techniques are suitable for analyzing data measured on ratio and interval scales [see Flannelly et al.'s (2014a) description in *JHCC of* different measurement scales].

Figure 5 illustrates six hypothetical sets of data (shown as circles, x's, and +'s) and their trend lines for the relationship between two variables, with one variable measured on the x axis and the other measured on the y axis. The three sets of data (and their trend lines) on the left side of Figure 5 all exhibit positive relationships between the two variables; larger values of the variable on the x axis are associated with larger values of the variable on the y axis. The three sets of data (and their trend lines) on the right side of Figure 5 all exhibit negative linear relationships between the two variables;

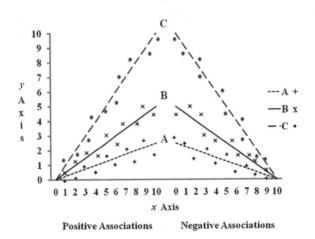

FIGURE 5 Trend lines depicting positive and negative linear associations between two variables.

larger values of the variable on the x axis are associated with smaller values of the variable on the y axis.

The slope of a trend line in OLS regression indicates the strength of the association. Hence, the two variables in the A datasets in Figure 5 have the weakest association with one another, regardless of the direction (positive or negative) of the relationship. The B dataset shows a stronger association between the two variables, regardless of direction, and the C dataset shows the strongest association between the variables, as indicted by the slope of the trend lines.

Selected examples of linear relationships in healthcare research include results from studies on the growth of palliative care programs in U.S. hospitals (Morrison, Maroney-Galin, Kralovec, & Meier, 2005), the increasing prevalence of fatty liver disease in U.S. adolescents (Welsh, Karpen, & Vos, 2013), the temporal changes in the prevalence rates of asthma in Australia (Ponsonby et al., 2008), and the incidence of breast cancer in Great Britain (Darbre, 2005). See Appendix 3 for more discussion of these examples.

Healthcare research often is designed to examine the relationship between categorical, also called nominal or qualitative, variables. The simplest example of this type of research compares the relative proportions of cases of a disease (an outcome variable) in relation to a variable that is thought to be a risk factor for the disease [see Flannelly et al. (2014b) explanation of independent, dependent, and other variables in healthcare research]. A 2×2 table, like Table 1, which the British mathematician Karl Pearson called a "contingency table" (David & Edwards, 2001), has long been a traditional method of presenting epidemiological observations (Fleiss, 1981).

Early studies of occupational health used retrospective cohort designs to study the effects of radiation and other toxic substances on the prevalence of cancer and other diseases among workers (Kelsey, Whitteman, Evans, & Thompson, 1996) [see the Flannelly and Jankowski (2014) article in *JHCC* describing epidemiological research designs]. These studies compared medical records from workers exposed to toxic substances, such as factory workers, to other workers in same industry who were not exposed to the toxic substances, such as office workers. Table 1 presents the hypothetical results of a retrospective cohort study of cancer among workers exposed to toxic

TABLE 1 Hypothetical Frequency and Percentage of Cases of Cancer Among Workers Who Were Exposed or Not Exposed to Toxic Substances at Work

	Exposed		Not exposed	
	n	%	n	%
Cancer	25	5	5	1
No Cancer	475	95	495	99
Total	500		500	

substances (e.g., benzene) used in the manufacturing of various products. The "observed" data indicate that 5% of the workers exposed to toxic substances at work were diagnosed with cancer, whereas only 1% of those who were not exposed were diagnosed with cancer.

The most common statistical test for evaluating the putative associations implied in a 2×2 table is the chi-square test, which we will explain in a later article. Suffice it to say for now that a chi-square test applied to the data in this example would confirm that the association between cancer and exposure to toxic substances at work is statistically significant.

More sophisticated statistical analyses employing another type of regression (i.e., logistic regression) can measure the strength of the association between the presence of a disease (case vs. no case) and the frequency, duration, and/or intensity of exposure to risk factors (Kahn & Sempos, 1989; Kleinbaum et al., 1998). Frequency in the current example might be how often a person worked in an area of the factory that contained toxic substances, duration might be number of years a person worked at the factory or plant, and intensity might be a measure of the level of toxic substances in the factory air.

CRITERIA FOR MAKING CAUSAL INFERENCES FROM ASSOCIATIONS

There is a "mantra" in science that "association does not imply causation." Causation can be difficult to determine in healthcare and other fields because an event (such as a disease) may have multiple causes. Logically, causes fall into two categories: necessary causes and sufficient causes (Copi, 1969). A necessary cause of an event "is a circumstance in whose absence the event cannot occur; a sufficient cause of an event "is a circumstance in whose presence the event must occur" (Copi, 1969, p. 322). Some causes may be both necessary and sufficient for an event to occur.

Though some viruses, such as rabies and measles, are necessary and sufficient to cause disease, whether an infectious agent results in disease usually depends on a number of factors, including age, genetic susceptibility, and other variables (Kelsey et al., 1996). Moreover, the sufficient cause of many diseases is not known, if one does exist (Kelsey et al., 1996). Given the multi-causality of disease, the identified causes of most diseases are not necessary or sufficient to produce disease (Rothman & Greenland, 2005). The problem of assigning causation led to the concept of risk factors. Coronary heart disease, for example, has many risk factors, including older age, being male, high blood pressure, high cholesterol, lack of exercise, and smoking, but none of these factors are necessary or sufficient to cause the disease (Kelsey et al., 1996). The problem of assigning causality also has led to the concept of "component causes" in which a "sufficient cause" is defined as "a set of minimal conditions and events that inevitably produce disease" (Rothman & Greenland, 2005). It is yet to be seen, however, if this definition of sufficient cause will be endorsed by researchers or clinicians.

Despite the fact that causation cannot be determined from "correlational" (i.e., nonexperimental) studies, researchers, much like the general public, are often inclined to imply causation from association. Hence, it should not be surprising to hear that some researchers have developed criteria for implying causal relationships between variables based on measures of association (e.g., Hill, 1965; Kelsey et al., 1996). The acclaimed British epidemiologist Sir Austin Bradford Hill proposed eight criteria for assessing causality from associations in 1965: (a) strength of association, (b) consistency, (c) specificity, (d) temporality, (e) biological gradient, (f) plausibility, (g) coherence, and (h) analogy (Hill, 1965). Though the utility and even the validity of Hill's criteria have been questioned (e.g., Hofler, 2005; Rothman & Greenland, 2005), they have been widely accepted (e.g., Katz, 2001; Kleinbaum, Kupper, & Morgenstern, 1982; Rothman & Greenland, 2005). Thus, we will briefly discuss them here.

Temporality

Although Hill (1965) listed temporality as his fourth criteria, we think it should be mentioned first because continuity in time has long been recognized to be central to causality (Hume, 1739/1896). Moreover, a temporal order in which a presumed cause precedes a presumed effect is critical for establishing a cause-effect relationship; from an epidemiological perspective, a disease should follow exposure to a disease agent (Kelsey et al., 1996). This is why prospective studies are better suited for helping to establish causal relationships than are retrospective studies; i.e., prospective studies can establish the temporal order between exposure and disease, whereas retrospective studies cannot do so (Flannelly & Jankowski, 2014; Kelsey et al., 1996). Indiscriminate reliance on temporality as evidence of causality, however, leads to the common logical fallacy of *post hoc ergo propter hoc*—after this, therefore, because of this.

Consistency

Hill's (1965) criterion of consistency also takes historical precedence over most of his other criteria, going back to the British philosopher John Stuart Mill's concept of "concomitant variation" between two variables as a sign of causality (Mill, 1859). Hill's (1965) concept of consistency was the extent to which an association was "repeatedly observed in different persons, in different places, circumstances and times" (p. 296). The criterion is useful because finding consistency only within similar groups or circumstances may indicate some unique feature of those groups or those circumstances rather than the nature of the association (Rothman & Greenland, 2005). Hill's use of the term persons is taken to mean different populations or different samples from a population. Inconsistent findings are as troublesome to experimental studies as they are to correlational studies. It is worth noting that inconsistent findings in both experimental and correlational studies may stem from differences in research methodology, including differences in sampling and measurement, which may obscure the underlying effects or associations.

Specificity

Hill's (1965) concept of specificity implied that a specific disease should have a specific cause. Therefore, one would expect that some putative cause would be related to a specific disease. However, he thought specificity could be problematic as a criterion of causality because diseases might have multiple causes and some events or circumstances (risk factors, as we now call them) might contribute to a number of diseases. Hill's criterion of specificity also dates back to John Stuart Mill (1859), but Mill's approach to determining the specificity of a cause-effect association between two variables was to develop experimental methods to determine if an apparent relationship was real (Copi, 1969; Mill, 1859). These methods have proven to be useful in many areas of science, including medicine, but they are of no use in epidemiology. Hill's approach to avoid the problem posed by specificity and multi-causality was to suggest that specificity should be used as a criterion in conjunction with strength of association.

Strength of Association

Hill probably placed strength of association first on his list because he thought it was the best evidence of causality aside from experimentation. He gave several examples of mortality rates as strong evidence of cause-effect relationships between behavior and disease, noting that prospective studies showed that the cancer mortality rate among cigarette smokers was 9 to 10 times higher than the rate among non-smokers. Some researchers have claimed that strength of association is a good index of causality because it indicates that the association between two variables is not the result of bias or other sources of error, or a third unknown variable (Kleinbaum et al., 1982; Kleinbaum et al., 1998; Rothman & Greenland, 2005). Measures of the strength of an association between two variables were developed, in part, by Karl Pearson near the end of the nineteenth century, including the statistical techniques of correlation and the chi-square test (David & Edwards, 2001; Pearson, 1920; Plackett, 1983).

Biological Gradient

Hill proposed that evidence of a dose-response relationship (or biological gradient) was indicative of a causal relationship. "For instance, the fact that the death rate from cancer of the lung rises linearly with the number of cigarettes smoked daily, adds a very great deal to the simpler evidence that cigarette smokers have a higher death rate than non-smokers" (Hill, 1965, p. 298). Kleinbaum et al. expressed this idea in a more general form: "The observation that the frequency of disease increases with the dose or level of exposure usually lends support to the causal interpretation" (Kleinbaum et al., 1982, p. 33). However, Hofler (2005) notes that Hill's and Kleinbaum et al.'s conception of a biological gradient implies that the association between two variables should be linear, even though the associations between health-related variables may not be linear.

Plausibility

Hill (1965) thought it was helpful if the causal relationship inferred from an association was biologically plausible, but recognized this was not always possible, especially given our limited knowledge of biology and medicine. Nevertheless, as Kleinbaum et al. (1982) state: "If the hypothesized effect makes sense in the context of current biological knowledge, we are more likely to accept a causal interpretation" (p. 34).

Coherence

On the other hand, Hill (1965) thought the possibility that an association indicates a cause-effect relationship should be considered to be less likely if it conflicts with what is known about the etiology of diseases. Kleinbaum and his colleagues express their agreement with this premise, which we paraphrase: Findings that do not seriously conflict with our knowledge of the natural history of disease should be more readily accepted as evidence of causality than findings that conflict with existing knowledge (Kleinbaum et al., 1982; Kleinbaum et al., 1998).

Analogy

Hill's (1965) last criterion for establishing a causal relationship between two variables by non-experimental means was by analogy, but he was very vague about how this could be done, saying, in essence, that knowledge about cause-effect relationships of one disease may be used to assess the probability of cause-effect relations in other diseases. Hill's statement has been interpreted to mean that when a class of factors has been demonstrated to have a casual effect on morbidity, the level of evidence required to establish that another agent in that class of factors has an effect on morbidity is lowered (Susser, 1991). However, as a paper critical of analogy as a criterion of causality stated: "Whatever insight might be derived from analogy is handicapped by the inventive imagination of scientists who can find analogies everywhere" (Rothman & Greenland, 2005, p. S149). Logically, as Copi

(1969) explains "Every analogical inference proceeds from the similarity of two or more things in one or more respects [the premise(s)] to the similarity of those things in some further respect [the inference]" (p. 307). Hence, the validity of the inference depends on the validity of the premise(s) that the things said to be similar are actually similar on some critical, relevant dimension(s). Researchers using analogy to identify a causal relationship must be especially clear in their description of variables, comparison of variables, and explanation of the relationships.

REFERENCES

Cajori, F. (1917). *A history of physics in its elementary branches.* New York, NY: Macmillan.

Chakrabarty, D. K. (2001). *An introduction to physical chemistry.* Pangbourne, UK: Alpha Science International.

Chen, C., Wang, J. C., Shi, Q., Zhou, W., Zhang, X. M., Zhang, J., ... Dong, X. P. (2013). Analyses of the survival time and the influencing factors of Chinese patients with prion diseases based on the surveillance data from 2008–2011. *PLoS ONE, 8*(5), e62553. doi:10.1371/journal.pone.0062553

Copi, I. M. (1969). *Introduction to logic* (3rd ed.). London, UK: MacMillan.

Darbre, P. D. (2005). Recorded quadrant incidence of female breast cancer in great britain suggests a disproportionate increase in the upper outer quadrant of the breast. *Anticancer Research, 25*(3C), 2543–2550.

David, H. A., & Edwards, A. W. F. (2001). *Annotated readings in the history of statistics.* New York, NY: Springer.

Flannelly, K. J., & Jankowski, K. R. B. (2014). Research designs and making causal inferences from health care studies. *Journal of Health Care Chaplaincy, 20*(1), 25–38. doi:10.1080/08854726.2014.871909

Flannelly, L. T., Flannelly, K. J., & Jankowski, K. R. B. (2014a). Fundamentals of measurement in health care research. *Journal of Health Care Chaplaincy, 20*(2), 75–82. doi:10.1080/08854726.2014.906262

Flannelly, L. T., Flannelly, K. J., & Jankowski, K. R. B. (2014b). Independent, dependent, and other variables in healthcare and chaplaincy research. *Journal of Health Care Chaplaincy, 20*(4), 161–170. doi:10.1080/08854726.2014.959374

Fleiss, J. L. (1981). *Statistical methods for rates and proportions* (2nd ed.). New York, NY: Wiley.

Gammelager, H., Christiansen, C., Johansen, M., Tonnesen, E., Jespersen, B., & Sorensen, H. (2012). One-year mortality among Danish intensive care patients with acute kidney injury: A cohort study. *Critical Care, 16*(4), R124. doi:10.1186/cc11420

Gibson, T. M., & Robison, L. L. (2015). Impact of cancer therapy-related exposures on late mortality in childhood cancer survivors. *Chemical Research in Toxicology, 28*(1), 31–37. doi:10.1021/tx500374k

Gong, Z., Lv, H., Ding, H., Han, J., Sun, J., Chai, C., ... Chen, E. (2014). Epidemiology of the avian influenza A (H7N9) outbreak in Zhejiang province, china. *BMC Infectious Diseases, 14*(244), 3–8. doi:10.1186/1471-2334-14-244

Guo, Z., Xiao, D., Li, D., Wang, X., Wang, Y., Yan, T., & Wang, Z. (2016). Predicting and evaluating the epidemic trend of Ebola virus disease in the 2014–2015 outbreak and the effects of intervention measures. *PLoS ONE, 11*(4), e0152438. doi:10.1371/journal.pone.0152438

Hill, A. B. (1965). The environment and disease: Association or causation? *Proceedings of the Royal Medical Society, 58,* 295–300.

Hofler, M. (2005). The Bradford hill considerations on causality: A counterfactual perspective. *Emerging Themes in Epidemiology, 2*(1), 1–9

Hume, D. (1739/1896). *A treatise of human nature.* Oxford, UK: The Clarendon Press.

Jordan, H., Fagliano, J., Rechtman, L., Lefkowitz, D., & Kaye, W. (2015). Effects of demographic factors on survival Time after a diagnosis of Amyotrophic lateral sclerosis. *Neuroepidemiology, 44*(2), 114–120. doi:10.1159/000380855

Kahn, H. A., & Sempos, C. T. (1989). *Statistical methods in epidemiology.* Oxford, UK: Oxford Univeristy Press.

Katz, D. L. (2001). *Clinical epidemiology & evidence-based medicine.* Thousand Oaks, CA: Sage Publications.

Kelsey, J., Whitteman, A. S., Evans, A. S., & Thompson, W. D. (1996). *Methods in observational epidemiology.* New York, NY: Oxford University Press.

Kleinbaum, D. G., Kupper, L. L., & Morgenstern, H. (1982). *Epidemiolic research: Principles and quantitative methods.* New York, NY: Van Nostrand Reinhold.

Kleinbaum, D. G., Kupper, L. L., Muller, K. E., & Nuzam, A. (1998). *Applied regression analysis and other multivariable methods.* Pacific Grove, CA: Duxbury Press.

Kumar, B. N. (2009). *Basic physics for all.* Lanham, MD: University Press of America.

Mill, J. S. (1859). *A system of logic, ratiocinative and inductive; bring a connected view of the principles of evidence and the methods of scientific investigation.* New York, NY: Harper & Brothers.

Morrison, R. S., Maroney-Galin, C., Kralovec, P. D., & Meier, D. E. (2005). The growth of palliative care programs in United States hospitals. *Journal of Palliative Medicine, 8*(6), 1127–1134. doi:10.1089/jpm.2005.8.1127

Pearson, K. (1920). Notes on the history of correlation. *Biometrika, 13*(1), 25–45. doi:10.1093/biomet/13.1.25

Plackett, R. L. (1983). Karl Pearson and the chi-squared test. *International Statistical Review, 51,* 59–72. doi:10.2307/1402731

Ponsonby, A. L., Glasgow, N., Pezic, A., Dwyer, T., Ciszek, K., & Kljakovic, M. (2008). A temporal decline in asthma but not eczema prevalence from 2000 to 2005 at school entry in the Australian capital territory with further consideration of country of birth. *International Journal of Epidemiology, 37*(3), 559–569. doi:10.1093/ije/dyn029

Rothman, K. J., & Greenland, S. (2005). Causation and causal inference in epidemiology. *American Journal of Public Health, 95*(51), S144–S150. doi:10.2105/ajph.2004.059204

Susser, M. (1991). What is a cause and how do we know one? A grammar for pragmatic epidemiology. *American Journal of Epidemiology, 133*(7), 635–648.

Welsh, J. A., Karpen, S., & Vos, M. B. (2013). Increasing prevalence of nonalcoholic fatty liver disease among United States adolescents, 1988–1994 to 2007–2010. *Journal of Pediatrics, 162*(3), 496–500.e1. doi:10.1016/j.jpeds.2012.08.043

APPENDIX 1: GRAPHS OF SURVIVAL RATES

The studies cited in Appendices 1–3 can be viewed and downloaded on PubMed for free. The Appendices use them as teaching tools to help the reader practice interpreting graphs that plot relationships with different shapes. For simplicity, all of the studies have graphs that show changes of a variable across time. To obtain the studies, go to http://www.ncbi.nlm.nih.gov/pubmed/, then copy the alpha- numeric code after the term "doi:" in the citation in the reference list, and paste it into the search window of PubMed.

As seen in the Chen et al. (2013) study, the survival rate of patients diagnosed with prion disease decreased rapidly during the first several months after diagnosis, with 50% surviving for just over seven months (Figure 2A). The slope of the curve became flatter after that, with some patients surviving until the 25th month post-diagnosis. Figure 1a of the Jordan et al. study indicates that approximately 50% of patients diagnosed with amyotrophic lateral sclerosis (Lou Gehrig's Disease) survived for the first 20 months after diagnosis, after which the curve was flatter, with survival decreasing up to 60 months. Figure 1c shows that the survival rates of the males and females in the study were comparable up to 16–17 months, with roughly 40% of both males and females surviving until then. After 16–17 months, the survival rates of males and females diverged, with males having a somewhat higher survival rate than females through 60 months.

APPENDIX 2: GRAPHS OF MORBIDITY AND MORTALITY RATES

Figure 2 of Gong et al. (2014) shows a roughly sigmoidal relationship (S-curve) in the cumulative number of cases, along with the underlying distribution of cases of a 2013 outbreak of avian flu over six months. Figure 3 of Guo et al. (2016) shows a classic S-curve of the cumulative number of cases of the Ebola virus during 14 months following a 2013 outbreak. The same figure shows that mortality followed a similar S-curve.

Figure 1 of the Gammelager et al. (2012) study presents four similar mortality curves for one year following kidney injuries during surgery. The curves differ in the rates of deaths, depending on the severity of the injury. Figure 3A of the Gibson and Robison (2015) study shows the mortality rate of childhood cancer patients over 30 years; approximately 50% died within 10 years of diagnosis, 60% died within 15 years, and 70% died within 20 years. While the death rate due to cancer showed a "concave" relationship, the rate from other causes showed a "convex" relationship with time.

APPENDIX 3: GRAPHS OF LINEAR ASSOCIATIONS

The top graph in Figure 1 of the Morrison et al. (2005) study shows a clear linear relationship in which a straight line is drawn in between four data points. Figure 2A of Welsh et al. (2013) illustrates (from top to bottom) a positive curvilinear trend, no change over time, and a positive linear trend. The results in Figure 1 of Ponsonby et al. (2008) are divided into three panels: Panel 1 depicts (from left to right) a moderate positive linear association and two moderate negative linear associations; Panel 2 displays a moderate negative linear association, and two graphs depicting no associations; Panel 3 contains three graphs depicting no linear association. The 2005 Darbre study is particularly helpful because it shows trend lines drawn between several series of data points, like those presented in our Figure 5. Figure 1 shows a moderate positive trend over time, whereas the top left and bottom right graphs in Figure 2 show substantial negative trends over time. The graph labeled "Upper Inner Quadrant" depicts a smaller negative association. The relatively flat lines shown in the remaining four graphs indicate that the variables do not change over time (i.e., they have no linear association with time).

The *t*-test: An Influential Inferential Tool in Chaplaincy and Other Healthcare Research

KATHERINE R. B. JANKOWSKI,KEVINJ.FLANNELLY
and LAURA T. FLANNELLY

The t-test developed by William S. Gosset (also known as Student's t-test and the two-sample t-test) is commonly used to compare one sample mean on a measure with another sample mean on the same measure. The outcome of the t-test is used to draw inferences about how different the samples are from each other. It is probably one of the most frequently relied upon statistics in inferential research. It is easy to use: a researcher can calculate the statistic with three simple tools: paper, pen, and a calculator. A computer program can quickly calculate the t-test for large samples. The ease of use can result in the misuse of the t-test. This article discusses the development of the original t-test, basic principles of the t-test, two additional types of t-tests (the one-sample t-test and the paired t-test), and recommendations about what to consider when using the t-test to draw inferences in research.

INTRODUCTION

"What kind of barley makes a better tasting beer?" This question appears to be unrelated to scientific methodology. Enjoying beer, or not enjoying it, is a matter of taste! Historically, brewing beer was a tradition-based endeavor. However, in the 1890s, Cecil Guinness and Christopher La Touche of the Guinness Brewing Company changed tradition by hiring chemists to identify what makes the best beer (Box, 1987). William S. Gosset, the man who is known for developing the *t*-test, was one of several chemists hired by Guinness. He, and the other chemists employed by Guinness, began methodically identifying the barley seeds that produced the best barley, and which of those produced the best beer.

It took years for the chemists to identify and measure the qualities of barley seeds associated with the best beer. Even after better seeds were identified, there was much variation in production. One batch of barley grown in one field would produce phenomenal barley while the same seed grown in a different field resulted in unsatisfactory barley. The chemists had to find a way to identify the best barley seed regardless of the variation that is due to things, such as a farmer's field, the weather, the manure used to fertilize it, and the maltster. Many years of planting specific kinds of barley in specific fields provided enough data for Gosset to calculate the average yield and the average amount of variation in the yield. He slowly worked out a mathematical equation to find the best seed and identified which seeds produced better beer than others, on average, even with the variation and the error that was inherent in their experimental research due to sampling and small sample size (Student, 1908). The *t*-test that is used today in scientific research was worked out mainly by Gosset, with some help from mathematicians Karl Pearson and Ronald A. Fisher (Boland, 1984; Box, 1987).

From the Seeds to the Table

The *t*-test that healthcare and other researchers use today has two parts: a mathematical equation that provides a number or value (the *t*-statistic), and a table of all the possible results of that equation (all possible *t*-statistics). The first part, the equation, is a mathematical way to represent the difference between one average (mean) and another number, which can be another average (mean) or a specific value, such as zero, taking into account the variability in the data (see explanation of the mean in Jankowski & Flannelly, 2015, and explanation of variability in K. J. Flannelly, Jankowski, & Flannelly, 2015). The second part, the table, is a standard table that lists all the possible mathematical outcomes of the *t*-test equation (*t*-statistics), and how likely each outcome is (also known as the probability of the outcome, the alpha level, *p* value, or critical value) given the sample size. As a result, the *t*-test is an equation that provides a value and a table that lists how likely that value is in the distribution of such values (the *t*-distribution, which is similar to the normal distribution).

A useful table of the critical values of the *t*-test does not list all of the possible numerical outcomes of the *t*-test equation because the table would be too large and not very helpful. What is helpful to researchers is knowing when the t-test equation produces an unlikely or unusual value of t (t-statistic). Today, computer programs do the calculations and provide the t-test equation result (the value of t) and the likelihood of that result (p) for a given sample size, which eliminates the need for an actual table of t values and their probability (p). Researchers, in general, agree that when the t-test result (the value of t) is unusual, when is expected to occur less than 5% of the time ($p < .05$), 1% of the time ($p < .01$), or less often (e.g., less than 1 time in 1,000; $p < .001$), the t-test result is statistically significant. Such unusual t-values support the inference that something is very different between the two means (or between a mean and zero) because the t-test result is not very likely to occur.

The t-test is based, in part, on the logic and mathematical proof of something called the Central Limit Theorem (Pagano, 2012). This theorem states that an entire population is well represented when a large enough sample is randomly drawn from it. In addition, any sample that is large enough and randomly drawn from a population will likely be similar to any other same-sized sample that is randomly drawn from the same population. Mathematically, it can be demonstrated that, if a researcher randomly pulled every possible same-size sample from a population, the means of all these same-size samples would produce a frequency bar graph that resembles a normal distribution or normal curve (the sampling distribution of the mean). Many of the means of the same-size samples would appear more frequently than others in the bar graph, and most would be near the population mean in the center of the curve. Some sample means would occur that are far away from the population mean and they would happen less frequently.

Similarly, the t-test equation produces a numerical outcome for a difference between sample means drawn from the same population (Pagano, 2012). A bar graph distribution of all possible t-test outcomes from all possible difference tests resembles a normal curve with larger sample sizes. A very unlikely t-test value indicates a very large difference between means and occurs away from the center of the bar graph in the tails of the distribution curve (see a description of the normal curve in K. J. Flannelly et al., 2015). In other words, a large difference between the sample means, relative to the variations in the data, yields a high t-value, which indicates that the difference between means is unusual and this allows for an inference that perhaps the samples are not from the same population.

TYPES OF t-TEST AND THEIR USES

There are three different but related types of t-tests, which are: (a) the two-sample or independent-samples t-test; (b) the matched- or paired t-test; and (c) the one-sample or single-sample t-test.

Two-Sample or Independent-Samples *t*-Test

The two-sample or independent samples *t*-test is based on the original *t*-test developed by Gossett. It is often called Student's *t*-test because Gosset published his article about it anonymously under the pseudonym Student (Boland, 1984; Box, 1987; Student, 1908). The two-sample *t*-test is used to compare the means of two samples to see if the difference is unusual and allow for the inference that the samples are not drawn from the same population. Two examples of studies that used two-sample *t*-tests, which we identified from a search of PubMed (see K. J. Flannelly, Jankowski, & Tannenbaum, 2011, about searching PubMed), tested the extent to which different treatment-team approaches improved patient care. One study assessed whether a multidisciplinary intervention improved the quality of life of advanced cancer patients, compared to standard care (Rummans et al., 2006), and the other study assessed the extent to which the implementation of an interdisciplinary care plan improved the end-of-life care of oncology and geriatric patients, compared to usual care (Bookbinder et al., 2005). A more recent study we found on PubMed used a two-sample *t*-test to compare spiritual well-being between samples of patients with generalized anxiety disorder and patients with minor general medical conditions (Ajman & Bokharey, 2015). Examples of articles published in the *Journal of Health Care Chaplaincy* (*JHCC*) include two studies that compared gender differences using two-sample *t*-tests. The first study examined sex differences in pastoral care skills among CPE (clinical pastoral education) students (Jankowski, Vanderwerker, Murphy, Montonye, & Ross, 2008) and the other study examined sex differences in the use of CAM (complementary alternative medical) practices by religious professionals (Jankowski, Silton, Galek, & Montonye, 2010). A third article reported the results of a national survey which found that healthcare chaplains who received workplace support had fewer symptoms of disenfranchised grief than those who did not receive workplace support (Spidell et al., 2011).

Paired or Dependent *t*-Test

The paired or dependent *t*-test is used to examine differences in means of two sets of data that are related to one another (hence, it is also called a correlated *t*-test). Typically, the paired *t*-test is used to compare the mean of a sample of people on a variable at two points in time.

The same type of *t*-test can be used with two samples if individuals in one sample are matched with those in another sample to form pairs based on their similarities on specific characteristics. This kind of matching procedure is mainly performed in epidemiological research (Jewell, 2004; Stewart, 2010; Stroup & Teutsch, 1998), where the paired *t*-test is sometimes referred to as a matched or matched-pairs *t*-test (Stroup & Teutsch, 1998).

The most common use of the paired t-test is to assess whether the scores of one sample of people on a scale or other measure have changed over time, as already noted. The paired t-test is widely used to examine the effects of an intervention (Katz, 2001) by comparing pretest (i.e., preintervention) and post-test (i.e., postintervention) scores on an *outcome* variable (also called a *dependent* variable, see L. T. Flannelly, Flannelly, & Jankowski, 2014b).

For example, we found two studies on PubMed that used paired t-tests to measure the effectiveness of educational programs, including the ability of educational programs to improve the ability of advanced medical students (von Gunten et al., 2012) and respiratory therapists to address end-of-life issues (Brown-Saltzman, Upadhya, Larner, & Wenger, 2010). Another study we found used paired t-tests to evaluate the health benefits of a religiously based wellness intervention (Kamieniski, Brown, Mitchell, Perrin, & Dindial, 2000),

There appear to be only two studies published in *JHCC* that used paired t-tests, one of which compared the ability of a faith-based chaplaincy intervention to reduce spiritual distress among patients at a U.S. Veteran Affairs Medical Center (Kopacz, Adams, & Searle, 2017). The other is a study that used both two-sample t-tests (as previously mentioned) and paired t-tests (Jankowski et al., 2008). The paired t-tests were used to assess changes between pretest and posttest scores on measures of pastoral skills, emotional intelligence, and self-reflection among CPE students (i.e., their scores before and after taking a unit of CPE).

One-Sample or Single-Sample t-Test

The one-sample or single-sample t-test is used to test one sample mean against a specific value, such as zero, or a standard or an expected outcome, or against the known population mean. If the t-test equation produces a t-value that is very unlikely, then the sample mean can be said to be significantly different from the standard mean, such as the normed average of a test. One-sample t-tests are often used to compare the mean of a sample of patients on some variable to the mean of the general population on that same variable.

No studies have ever been published in *JHCC* that used a one-sample t-test, but we found several interesting studies on PubMed that used it. For example, two recent studies compared the mean of the post-op quality of life of surgical patients in the United States and Italy to the quality of life of the general population in their respective countries (Schiavolin et al., 2015; Steele, Zahr, Kirshbom, Kopf, & Karimi, 2016). Similarly, a Dutch study used a one-sample t-test to compare the perceptions of diabetes patients about their state of health to the perceived health of the general population of The Netherlands (Hart, Redekop, Bilo, Berg, & Meyboom-de Jong, 2005).

The reader may think it is odd that this kind of t-test is called a single-sample or a one-sample t-test, as two means are being compared. However, the term one-sample is based on the fact that the mean of one sample is compared to an accepted standard mean value. In the case of these three studies, the standard to which the sample mean is compared is the mean of the general population.

CONSIDERATIONS LENDING CONFIDENCE TO INFERENCES

Sample Considerations

When using a t-test, it is important that the sample of data has 30 data points or more because a sample size of thirty or more will more closely resemble the population and the sampling distribution of the mean of the normal distribution (Triola, 2004). This relates directly to the Central Limit Theorem. A larger sample size helps the researcher have greater confidence that the sample average and variation in the data, closely reflect the population average and variation, unless there is truly something different in the sample due to treatment or other influences. A larger sample size is also needed to detect smaller differences in means (effect sizes). Random sampling from the population is assumed, meaning that the data used for the t-test come from a random selection of participants from a larger population. In random sampling, everyone has an equal chance to be selected for the study, and it is also important that everyone has an equal chance to be included in any group in the study (random assignment).

Data Considerations

The data used to calculate the t-test must be on at least an interval scale. Ideally, the measurement should provide data that range across at least 11 values (see L. T. Flannelly, Flannelly, & Jankowski, 2014a, for examples of interval and ratio scales). The data must be free from extreme values, also known as outliers. Outliers are found when some participants in a study have scores on a measure that are extremely different from the scores of everyone else. Outliers can be found by arranging all the data in ascending or descending order, or by creating a bar graph. The t-test should not be used with outliers in the data because outliers affect the mean and standard deviation, and thereby, affect the accuracy of the t-test results. Also, attention should be given to the shape of the distribution of the data by charting the data in a bar graph. The distribution of data in the sample should be balanced around the average of the data in the sample, and there should be only one mode. A distribution of data in this shape, often referred to as a normal distribution or normal curve, can be seen in the distribution of pain scores in K. J. Flannelly et al. (2015; Figure 1). Work by Poncet, Courvoisier, Combescure, and

Perneger (2016) suggests, that in some situations, lack of normality might not negatively affect the interpretation of *t*-test results as dramatically as was once thought.

Reporting and Interpreting the *t*-Test Outcomes

Always report the *t*-test value, the degrees of freedom, and the probability of the observed outcome (*p* value). The degrees of freedom refer to the sample size minus one. It is also important to report the means and standard deviations for the samples tested by the *t*-test. This helps the reader understand and evaluate the results of the *t*-test. It is also becoming accepted practice to report the effect size (Cohen's d; Cohen, 1988), which is the difference between the two means divided by the standard deviation of the combined samples (see the explanation and calculation of the standard deviation in K. J. Flannelly et al., 2015).

Interpretation of the *t*-test result is guided by the probability (*p* value) of the outcome (*t* statistic). If the probability is very small, a researcher can conclude that the difference between sample means is unusual. The *t*-test does not prove anything. It indicates the probability of obtaining the observed difference between the means. When the result is significant, the *t*-test indicates that the outcome happens 5.0%, 2.5%, or 1.0% of the time, or even less often. It is up to the researcher to infer from all of the information regarding the samples if there is truly an important difference between two samples and what that difference means. The *t*-test result is just the beginning to understanding the story of what is being studied.

Interpretation of *t*-test results should also be guided by how many *t*-tests are calculated on the same data. If many *t*-tests are being calculated on the same data it is customary to reduce the critical level for the *t*-test, also known as the alpha level, or *p* level, by dividing the usual .05 by the number of *t*-tests conducted (Gordon, 2012).

Finally, it must always be kept in mind that the results from a single *t*-test in a single study are just the beginning. Science moves forward best by replication of findings, and this means doing more than one study. A similar, second study of the same variables may not necessarily produce the same finding. There is serious difficulty with scientists not being able to replicate the findings of studies, and whole theories built on a single finding might not be supported by further research (see Pashler & Wagenmakers, 2012, for a cautionary tale and Pashler & Harris, 2012, for a fuller explanation of the interpretation of $p < .05$). There are a number of reasons for this recent lack of replication, but going back to the basic understanding of the Central Limit Theorem, some studies might not find similar results because the original results, differences between groups identified by the *t*-test, might just have been due to the fact that the differences observed in means can occur in the same population, just not very often.

CONCLUSIONS

The *t*-test is a go-to statistic that can be used to test a difference between the mean of a sample with the mean of another sample or a standard mean. The *t*-test is easy to use and easy to use incorrectly. The test provides information on whether means are different from one another, provided that certain conditions are met, such as random sampling and a reasonable sample size. The test provides a statistical window to look through to see if the difference observed between two means is notably unusual, occurring 5% of the time or much less. A significant *t*-test result leads to inferences about what the research results might mean, encourages further investigation, and may be the beginning of a new research story.

REFERENCES

Ajman, F., & Bokharey, I. Z. (2015). Comparison of spiritual well-being and coping strategies of patients with generalized anxiety disorder and with minor general medical conditions. *Journal of Religion and Health, 54*(2), 524–539. doi:10.1007/s10943-014-9834-2

Boland, P. J. (1984). A biographical glimpse of William Sealy Gosset. *The American Statistician, 38*(3), 179–183. doi:10.1080/00031305.1984.10483195

Bookbinder, M., Blank, A. E., Arney, E., Wollner, D., Lesage, P., McHugh, M., ... Portenoy, R. K. (2005). Improving end-of-life care: Development and pilot-test of a clinical pathway. *Journal of Pain and Symptom Management, 29*(6), 529–543. doi:10.1016/j.jpainsymman.2004.05.011

Box, J. F. (1987). Guinness, Gosset, Fisher, and small samples. *Statistical Science, 2*(1), 45–52. doi:10.1214/ss/1177013437

Brown-Saltzman, K., Upadhya, D., Larner, L., & Wenger, N. S. (2010). An intervention to improve respiratory therapists' comfort with end-of-life care. *Respiratory Care, 55*(7), 858–865.

Cohen, J. (1988). *Statistical power analysis for the behavioral sciences* (2nd ed.). Hillside, NJ: Lawrence Erlbaum.

Flannelly, K. J., Jankowski, K. R. B., & Flannelly, L. T. (2015). Measures of variability in chaplaincy, health care, and related research. *Journal of Health Care Chaplaincy, 21*(3), 122–130. doi:10.1080/08854726.2015.1054671

Flannelly, K. J., Jankowski, K. R. B., & Tannenbaum, H. P. (2011). Keys to knowledge: Searching and reviewing the literature relevant to chaplaincy. *Chaplaincy Today, 27*(1), 10–15. doi:10.1080/10999183.2011.10767418

Flannelly, L. T., Flannelly, K. J., & Jankowski, K. R. B. (2014a). Fundamentals of measurement in health care research. *Journal of Health Care Chaplaincy, 20*(2), 75–82. doi:10.1080/08854726.2014.906262

Flannelly, L. T., Flannelly, K. J., & Jankowski, K. R. B. (2014b). Independent, dependent, and other variables in healthcare and chaplaincy research. *Journal of Health Care Chaplaincy, 20*(4), 161–170. doi:10.1080/08854726.2014.959374

Gordon, R. A. (2012). *Applied statistics for the social and health sciences.* New York, NY: Routledge.

Hart, H. E., Redekop, W. K., Bilo, H. J., Berg, M., & Meyboom-de Jong, B. (2005). Change in perceived health and functioning over time in patients with type I diabetes mellitus. *Quality of Life Research, 14*(1), 1–10. doi:10.1007/s11136-004-0782-2

Jankowski, K. R. B., & Flannelly, K. J. (2015). Measures of central tendency in chaplaincy, healthcare, and related research. *Journal of Health Care Chaplaincy, 21*(1), 39–49. doi:10.1080/08854726.2014.989799

Jankowski, K. R. B., Silton, N. R., Galek, K., & Montonye, M. G. (2010). Complementary alternative medicine practices used by religious professionals. *Journal of Health Care Chaplaincy, 16*(3–4), 172–182. doi:10.1080/08854726.2010.498694

Jankowski, K. R. B., Vanderwerker, L. C., Murphy, K. M., Montonye, M., & Ross, A. M. (2008). Change in pastoral skills, emotional intelligence, self-reflection, and social desirability across a unit of CPE. *Journal of Health Care Chaplaincy, 15*(2), 132–148. doi:10.1080/08854720903163304

Jewell, N. P. (2004). *Statistics for epidemiology.* New York, NY: Chapman & Hall/CRC.

Kamieniski, R., Brown, C. M., Mitchell, C., Perrin, K. M., & Dindial, K. (2000). Health benefits achieved through the Seventh-Day Adventist wellness challenge program. *Alternative Therapies in Health and Medicine, 6*(6), 65–69.

Katz, D. L. (2001). *Clinical epidemiology & evidence based medicine.* Thousand Oaks, CA: Sage.

Kopacz, M. S., Adams, M. S., & Searle, R. F. (2017). Lectio Divina: A preliminary evaluation of a chaplaincy program. *Journal of Health Care Chaplaincy, 23*(3), 87–97. doi:10.1080/08854726.2016.1253263

Pagano, R. P. (2012). *Understanding statistics in the behavioral sciences* (10th ed.). Belmont, CA: Wadsworth.

Pashler, H., & Harris, C. R. (2012). Is the replicability crisis overblown? Three arguments examined. *Perspectives on Psychological Science, 7*(6), 531–536. doi:10.1177/1745691612463401

Pashler, H., & Wagenmakers, E. J. (2012). Editors' introduction to the special section on replicability in psychological science: A crisis of confidence? *Perspectives on Psychological Science, 7*(6), 528–530. doi:10.1177/1745691612465253

Poncet, A., Courvoisier, D. S., Combescure, C., & Perneger, T. V. (2016). Normality and sample size do not matter for the selection of an appropriate statistical test for two-group comparisons. *Methodology, 12*(2), 61–71. doi:10.1027/1614-2241/a000110

Rummans, T. A., Clark, M. M., Sloan, J. A., Frost, M. H., Bostwick, J. M., Atherton, P. J., … Hanson, J. (2006). Impacting quality of life for patients with advanced cancer with a structured multidisciplinary intervention: A randomized controlled trial. *Journal of Clinical Oncology, 24*(4), 635–642. doi:10.1200/jco.2006.06.209

Schiavolin, S., Broggi, M., Visintini, S., Schiariti, M., Leonardi, M., & Ferroli, P. (2015). Change in quality of life, disability, and well-being after decompressive surgery: Results from a longitudinal study. *International Journal of Rehabilitation Research, 38*(4), 357–363. doi:10.1097/mrr.0000000000000136

Spidell, S., Wallace, A., Carmack, C. L., Nogueras-González, G. M., Parker, C. L., & Cantor, S. B. (2011). Grief in healthcare chaplains: An investigation of the presence of disenfranchised grief. *Journal of Health Care Chaplaincy, 17*(1–2), 75–86. doi:10.1080/08854726.2011.559859

Steele, M. M., Zahr, R. A., Kirshbom, P. M., Kopf, G. S., & Karimi, M. (2016). Quality of life for historic cavopulmonary shunt survivors. *World Journal for Pediatric and Congenital Heart Surgery, 7*(5), 630–634. doi:10.1177/2150135116658009

Stewart, A. (2010). *Basic statistics and epidemiology: A practical guide* (3rd ed.). New York, NY: Radcliffe.

Stroup, D. F., & Teutsch, S. M. (Eds.) (1998). *Statistics in public health: Quantitative approaches to public health problems.* New York, NY: Oxford University Press.

Student. (1908). The probable error of a mean. *Biometrika, 6*(1), 1–25. doi:10.1093/biomet/6.1.1

Triola, M. F. (2004). *Elementary statistics* (2nd ed.). Boston, MA: Pearson.

von Gunten, C. F., Mullan, P., Nelesen, R. A., Soskins, M., Savoia, M., Buckholz, G., & Weissman, D. E. (2012). Development and evaluation of a palliative medicine curriculum for third-year medical students. *Journal of Palliative Medicine, 15*(11), 1198–1217. doi:10.1089/jpm.2010.0502

Threats to the Internal Validity of Experimental and Quasi-Experimental Research in Healthcare

KEVIN J. FLANNELLY, LAURA T. FLANNELLY
andKATHERINER.B.JANKOWSKI

The article defines, describes, and discusses the seven threats to the internal validity of experiments discussed by Donald T. Campbell in his classic 1957 article: history, maturation, testing, instrument decay, statistical regression, selection, and mortality. These concepts are said to be threats to the internal validity of experiments because they pose alternate explanations for the apparent causal relationship between the independent variable and dependent variable of an experiment if they are not adequately controlled. A series of simple diagrams illustrate three pre-experimental designs and three true experimental designs discussed by Campbell in 1957 and several quasi-experimental designs described in his book written with Julian C. Stanley in 1966. The current article explains why each design controls for or fails to control for these seven threats to internal validity.

INTRODUCTION

Claude Bernard, the father of experimental medicine, proposed that experimentation was needed in medicine to help physicians "conserve health and cure disease" (Bernard, 1865/1957, p. 1), by providing knowledge about the causes of normal states of health (i.e., anatomy and physiology), the causes of disease (i.e., pathology), and the effectiveness of therapeutic treatments. Bernard's 1865 book, *An Introduction to the Study of Experimental Medicine,* emphasized the difference between the simple observation of natural changes in physiological processes over the course of time and experimentation, in which the researcher intervenes in some way to change the natural course of physiological processes. There are four important stages in the research process according to Bernard. The researcher (a) observes a natural phenomenon, (b) develops a hypothesis about the phenomenon, (c) applies a procedure to test this hypothesis, and (d) compares the results before and after applying the procedure.

Six years earlier, the philosopher John Stuart Mill (1859) published a book that laid out the principles he mainly developed for inferring causality from research results. The first principle was that the putative or presumed cause must occur before the effect. The second was that the effect must always occur when the presumed cause occurs. Third, the effect must not occur when the presumed cause is absent. Fourth, the presumed cause must be isolated from other potential causes of the effect. Fifth, the presumed cause must be produced artificially to ensure that the cause is isolated from all other potential causes. These principles set the standard for establishing casual relationships between presumed causes and effects (see K. J. Flannelly & Jankowski, 2014a). The fourth and fifth principles distinguish experimentation from other forms of research in that the experimenter must be able to manipulate the presumed cause and isolate the effects of the presumed cause from other events or variables (i.e., see discussion of variables by L. T. Flannelly, Flannelly, & Jankowski, 2014a) that could cause the observed effect.

Based on Mill's (1859) principles, an experimenter tries to control or hold constant all the variables that can affect the outcome (the dependent variable) of an experiment apart from the experimental manipulation (Keppel & Wickens, 2004), which is also called the independent variable, intervention, or treatment (see L. T. Flannelly et al., 2014a). The variables that the researcher wants to control are known as both extraneous variables, because they are extraneous to the purpose of the experiment, and confounding variables, because their effects are confounded with the effects of the independent variable if they are not properly controlled. The explicit concern is that "the operation of some extraneous variable causes the observed values of the dependent variable to inaccurately reflect the effect of the independent variable" (Cherulnik, 1983, p. 21). In other words, the observed effect of the experiment is not due to the independent variable, but to the extraneous variable. Thus, the failure to control extraneous variables undermines the ability of researchers to logically make the causal inference that the apparent effect of an experimental manipulation is, in fact, the result of the manipulation (i.e., the independent variable or intervention). Unfortunately, it is not very easy to control extraneous variables outside of a laboratory setting (Rubinson & Neutens, 1987).

Donald T. Campbell published a classic article in 1957 that describes the types or classes of extraneous variables a researcher must control in order to be able to make causal inferences from an experiment. He also explains why causal inferences cannot be made from various types of experimental designs. Campbell called the degree to which a design controls extraneous variables and, thus, permits causal inferences to be made regardiing the association between the independent and dependent variable, the experiment's "internal validity." An experiment with a high degree of internal validity has reduced the potential influence of extraneous variables to such an extent that the independent variable is the most likely cause of the observed change in the dependent variable. An experiment with low internal validity has not eliminated the possibility that some variable other than the independent variable has caused the observed change in the dependent variable. Even though Campbell's article is titled "Factors Relevant to the Validity of Experiments in Social Settings," it is applicable to all experimentation involving human participants.

Campbell's (1957) article focuses on seven classes of extraneous variables that can undermine the internal validity of an experiment if they are not controlled by the experimental design of a study. Thus, these classes of extraneous variables are called "threats to internal validity." Campbell named them: *history, maturation, testing, instrument decay, statistical regression, selection,* and *mortality*. Properly controlling for these variables eliminates them as rival explanations for the results of an experiment. Campbell also discussed factors that affect the "external validity" or generalizability of an experiment's results, but we will not address them in this article.

Campbell's (1957) analysis of the threats to internal validity posed by different designs was extended in his later writings that expanded from pre-experimental and experimental designs to include what he called quasi-experimental designs (Campbell & Stanley, 1966; Cook & Campbell, 1979), which are discussed later. Although the concepts of internal validity and threats to the internal validity of experimental designs are briefly summarized in some books on healthcare research (e.g., Kane, 2005; Keele, 2012; Rubinson & Neutens, 1987; Tappan, 2015), a search of PubMed found they have received minimal attention in medical or other healthcare journals despite the fact that randomized controlled trials (RCTs), which are true experiments, are considered to be the "gold standard" of medical research

(Greenhalgh, 2001; Salmond, 2008). Campbell and Stanley's "Experimental and Quasi-Experimental Designs for Research" is a particularly valuable resource for understanding internal validity and external validity and it can be downloaded from the Internet for free. Explanations of the seven threats to internal validity are given in the following sections.

SEVEN THREATS TO THE INTERNAL VALIDITY OF EXPERIMENTS

History

Campbell's (1957) concept of *history* might be called experience, but *history* in the Campbell conception of threats to internal validity specifically encompasses those things (i.e., specific events) that a study participant experiences during the course of an experiment that are not part of the experiment itself; therefore, they are extraneous variables. In hospital settings, history may include the transfer of patients between units, staff assignment changes, symptom exacerbation, and adverse events associated with treatments. If an experiment takes only a few minutes, *history* is not likely to be a threat to internal validity. Even if an experiment takes a few hours, *history* may not be a threat to internal validity if the study involves hospitalized patients whose experience is limited by the confines of a hospital. However, many experiments may be conducted over, days, weeks, or months. Thus, common everyday experiences like reading or listening to news stories may affect study outcomes. While it may be unlikely that news stories will affect physiological measures of study participants' responses to a medical treatment for cancer, diabetes, or some other medical problem, they are likely to affect psychological outcome measures if the patients learn a new medical treatment is improving health outcomes for these medical ailments or learn that some new treatment has fallen short of its expected efficacy. Participants' outcomes may also be affected by the extent to which they communicate their personal experiences, including perceived treatment effects, with other participants in a study.

Maturation

Whereas *history* involves the experience of external events, *maturation* involves bodily changes. The concept of *maturation* in the context of internal validity encompasses much more than the processes we usually think of as *maturation,* like age-related biological changes. It also encompasses any biological changes that occur with the passage of time, such as becoming hungry, tired, or fatigued, wound healing, recovering from surgery, and disease progression (e.g., stages of cancer or other diseases). Fatigue can occur even during brief interventions with young children, elderly persons, and patients who are feeling ill.

Taylor and Asmundson (2008) provide a hypothetical example of a study in which *maturation* presents a threat to internal validity because the study does not control for it. The example is a "single arm study"[1] of older adults in the early stages of Alzheimer's disease who showed improvement in depression after being treated with a new antidepressant medication. The researchers concluded that the participants' improved mood was due to the medication, when in fact, the depression of many of the participants had remitted naturally as their dementia progressed. As their memory declined, their awareness and insight into their dementia decreased, and they were no longer depressed about the problem.

Testing

The term *testing* is shorthand for any form of measuring study outcomes in study participants. These include physiological measures, which range from having their blood pressure and temperature taken to undergoing an MRI (magnetic resonance imaging). Behavioral tests include such tasks as answering questions on a survey, taking an eye test, or taking a psychological test. Since health researchers often measure a health outcome (the dependent variable) before and after treatment, *testing* becomes a threat to internal validity if the test itself can affect participants' responses when they are tested again. Campbell (1957) called such a test a "reactive measure." This can happen when the test measures participants' knowledge regarding a topic and they learn the correct answers to the questions before taking the test again. It could also happen when a test measures participants' attitudes about a topic and they alter their responses when tested again to give more socially acceptable answers to questions. However, deceit is not the only type of problem posed by repeated testing. The initial test may make some study participants more attuned to the health outcome of interest in a study. An initial measure of personal dietary habits might make a study participant think about his or her poor eating habits and improve them during the course of the study. Similarly, an initial measure of personal exercise might increase a study participant's awareness of his or her lack of exercise and increase how much s/he exercises over the course of the study. These actions would pose threats to the internal validity of experiments designed to improve diet and exercise, respectively, if this participant was in the control group of those experiments; that is, the group of participants who did not receive the intervention.

Measures or tests are less likely to be reactive when they are part of a regular routine, such as measures of temperature, blood pressure, heart rate, and other standard tests patients undergo during their hospital stay. Therefore, the degree to which a researcher can incorporate a measure of the health outcome of interest into the study participants' usual routine, the less likely the measure is to be reactive and, therefore, the less likely it is to pose a threat to the internal validity of an experiment (Campbell, 1957; Campbell & Stanley, 1966).

Campbell (1957) suggests that a good way to reduce the reactivity of a measure is to embed it in an array of other measures, especially measures that may distract participants from the focus of the study. Unobtrusive observation of patient behavior and reviews of patient charts are nonreactive measures that are very useful if they are applicable to the research question. Webb, Campbell, Schwartz, and Sechrest (1966) discussed the value of observational, archival, and other nonreactive measures in their 1966 book (*Unobtrusive Measures*) and later editions of the book that are still available.

Instrument Decay

Campbell's (1957) concept of *instrument decay* is exemplified by a researcher using a battery-powered device to measure blood pressure in an experiment investigating the effectiveness of a drug to reduce hypertension. Consider an experiment designed for the researcher to measure the blood pressure of the participants before (a "pretest") and after (a "posttest") the participants take the drug for one month. Suppose, however, that unbeknownst to the researcher, the battery has decayed during the month so all the blood-pressure readings taken by the device are lower on the posttest than they were on the pretest.[2] This would severely undermine the internal validity of the experiment. One can imagine a similar experiment to evaluate the effectiveness of a drug to reduce anxiety, in which the researcher assessed anxiety using two battery-powered devices to measure galvanic-skin-response (GSR), a common physiological measure of anxiety. Further imagine that the researcher used one device to measure the GSR of the participants in the experimental group (the participants who took the drug for a month) and the second device to measure the GSR of the participants in the control group (the participants who did not take the drug). If the battery decayed in the device used with experimental participants but not in the device used with control participants, the GSR readings would, hypothetically, be lower for the experimental group than the control group. This would lead the researcher to conclude that the drug reduced anxiety, when, in fact, the observed effect was due to the faulty battery, not the drug.

Campbell and Stanley (1966) changed the term *instrument decay* to *instrumentation* to reflect the fact that any change in measurement ability can pose a threat to internal validity. The term instrument, as used by Campbell (1957) and Campbell and Stanley (1966) is not limited to electronic or mechanical instruments, and applied to any means of measuring the dependent variable, including human researchers or research assistants who observe, judge, rate, and/or otherwise measure a dependent variable. For instance, suppose a new medical resident at an out-patient clinic receives training to observe and rate the functional health-status of patients who volunteered for a study, using the 0 to 100 Karnofsky Performance Scale (KPS) (e.g., Crooks, Waller, Smith, & Hahn, 1991; Terret, Albrand, Moncenix, & Droz, 2011).[3] After the training, the resident rates all the patients in the study as the pretest, after which half the patients receive a one-month intervention to improve their level of functioning. Because the resident regularly works at the clinic, he becomes better at observing patients and using the KPS by the time he performs the patient ratings for the posttest. This change in *instrumentation* undermines the study's internal validity. A similar problem would arise if someone with extensive experience using the KPS left the research team and had to be replaced with someone new. Since all observers probably get better at observing the more they do it, researcher assistants or other observers on a research team must be thoroughly trained before the start of an experiment.

Statistical Regression

Statistical regression is the tendency for individuals who score extremely high or extremely low, relative to the mean or average, on an initial measure of a variable to score closer to the mean of that variable the next time they are measured on it. *Statistical regression* is more accurately referred to as *regression toward the mean*. It is a threat to internal validity because individuals who are selected for a study because they score high on some measure are likely to score lower on that measure the next time they are tested even without an experimental intervention, whereas individuals who are selected for a study because they score low on some measure are likely to score higher on that measure the next time they are tested even without any experimental intervention (Campbell, 1957; Campbell & Stanley, 1966). Thus, if participants are selected for very low scores on some measure, such as a pretest of reading comprehension, and given an intervention to improve their comprehension of what they read, they are likely to score higher on the posttest even without the intervention to improve their reading comprehension.

An example would be a hospital that wanted to increase its medical interns' awareness of end-of-life issues (e.g., advance directives) and, therefore, might want to offer an in-service. The hospital might decide it would be more efficient to give the in-service only to those interns who seemed to need it the most. As a result, it gave all the interns a test regarding end-of-life issues and selected those who scored the lowest to attend the in-service, and test them after the in-service to see if their scores improved. Since test scores are affected by many things in addition to the knowledge regarding a topic, some interns might have scored very low on the initial test because they were not motivated, they felt tired, they were upset about something that had happened earlier during the day of the test, or were distracted by things that they had to do later that day. Hence, their scores might have increased when they were tested again, even if they had not attended the in-service.

The concept of *statistical regression* or, more precisely, *regression toward the mean* may seem odd or esoteric, but it is quite common, as sports fans should recognize. Although a few teams in any sport may consistently perform better than or worse than the average team, in terms of the number of games they win each year, most teams are always closer to the average, and the teams who do extremely better or worse than average in one year are likely to be closer to the average the next year.

Selection

Selection refers to a potential bias in selecting the participants who will serve in the experimental and control groups; hence it is also known as *selection bias*. The threat to internal validity is that the individuals who are assigned to the experimental and control groups differ from each other in some important ways; that is, that the groups are not equivalent. *Selection bias* would be an obvious problem if participants were allowed to choose whether they participated in the control group or the experimental group (i.e., self-selection), but *selection bias* is usually more subtle. For example, a researcher might decide to assign patients at a hemodialysis (HD) center to the experimental and control groups of a study to improve patients' quality-of-life, based on the days of the week they receive treatment [e.g., Monday, Wednesday, and Friday (MWF) vs. Tuesday, Thursday, and Saturday (TTS)]. Although this may seem like a good approach, the patients receiving HD treatment on the MWF schedule probably differ in a number of ways from those receiving it on the TTS schedule. Indeed, the fact that they chose different treatment schedules probably reflects some of these differences; therefore, these differences are confounded with the effects of a quality-of-life intervention, which would undermine the study's internal validity.

Another example of *selection bias* is provided by a hypothetical experiment in which a researcher wants to test the effectiveness of an 8-week family-based, weight-loss program for obese elementary school children. After obtaining permission for the study from the school board and school principals, and distributing flyers regarding the study to parents, the parents begin to enroll their families to participate in the experiment. As the experimental condition is more time-consuming for the researcher to conduct than the control condition is, he decides to "run" the experimental condition (i.e., implement the experimental intervention) first, while he has the time, and run the control condition after the experimental condition is done. Hence, he assigns all the families who immediately enroll in the program to the experimental group, and subsequent families to the control group. Because this decision biases the selection of the participants for the two groups (*selection bias*), the results of the experiment may reflect differences in the families assigned to the experimental and control groups, rather than the effectiveness of the experimental treatment. One such difference might be that the parents who immediately enrolled their families in the study were more motivated to reduce their child's weight than were the parents who enrolled their families later.

Mortality

Campbell's (1957) *mortality* (sometimes called *experimental mortality*) refers to the differential loss of study participants in the experimental and control groups. This loss is more commonly referred to as the *drop-out rate,* or simply *attrition.* The *drop-out rate* is more likely to be higher for an experimental group than a control group because experimental procedures usually make more demands on and require more commitment and effort from participants. If less committed individuals drop-out of the experimental group, the results may suggest that the intervention is more beneficial than it actually is. For example, individuals who exercise regularly or want to exercise regularly are more likely than other individuals in the experimental group to complete an exercise intervention that lasts several weeks. Thus, results indicating that the experimental intervention was superior to the control condition would be based on a selective subgroup of the original experimental group, and the selective subgroup may be more likely to benefit from the intervention because of their greater motivation to exercise.

INTERNAL VALIDITY OF THREE PRE-EXPERIMENTAL DESIGNS

Campbell described three of what he called pre-experimental designs (Campbell, 1957; Campbell & Stanley, 1966). The three designs are illustrated in Figures 1–3, using the symbols they used to denote the observation or measurement of the dependent variable (**O**) and the presentation of the independent variable (**X**), also referred to as an intervention or treatment.

One-Shot Case Study

Figure 1 shows that this design consists of a single group of participants who receive an intervention (**X**), which is followed by some measure of the dependent variable (**O**). Campbell (1957) said "This design does not merit the title of an experiment" and that he only included it as "a reference point" (p. 298). Fred Kerlinger (1973), who wrote several books regarding research, claimed this design has no scientific value, although he seemed to concede it has clinical value. We think it also has some utility in the context of education,

Group   X   O

FIGURE 1 One-shot case study.

although it obviously does not control for *history* or *maturation* because it lacks a control group. Hence, there is no way of knowing whether the observed value of the dependent variable is due to the independent variable.

Moreover, the lack of a pretest means there is no way of knowing if the value of the dependent variable was any different after the independent variable was introduced than it was before the independent variable was introduced. The other threats to internal validity do not come into play because of the simplicity of the design.

A study submitted to the *Journal of Health Care Chaplaincy* (*JHCC*) several years ago attempted to use this design to demonstrate that satisfaction with chaplaincy services among the staff of several hospital departments increased after the chaplaincy department made changes to better integrate its services with the services provided by those departments (the study's independent variable). The study was rejected for publication because the authors claimed that staff satisfaction with the chaplaincy department improved after the changes were made without conducting a pretest to measure staff satisfaction with the chaplaincy department before the changes were made; thus, the study could not provide evidence of an improvement in staff satisfaction after the changes were made.

However, *JHCC* has published four articles employing the same design in what are called program description and evaluation studies, which are consistent with the pre-experimental nature of this design. The first article evaluated a curriculum for chaplaincy residents to increase their research skills (Derrickson & Van Hise, 2010), and the last article evaluated a journal club to increase the research skills of chaplaincy residents (Fleenor, Sharma, Hirschmann, & Swarts, 2017). The second one evaluated a curriculum on spiritual assessment for chaplaincy, social work, and medical students (Lennon-Dearing, Florence, Halvorson, & Pollard, 2012), and the third one evaluated a chaplaincy residency program in palliative care (Jackson-Jordan et al., 2017). The four studies had the program participants provide feedback regarding the personal and professional value of the program, the program's implementation (e.g., were program goals clear and were they met), and ways to improve it.

One-Group Pretest-Posttest Design

Figure 2 depicts Campbell's (1957) One-Group Pretest–Posttest Design. The design consists of one group of participants who are given a pretest to measure the dependent variable (O_1), followed by an intervention (X), and a posttest to measure the dependent variable again (O_2).

$$\textbf{Group} \quad \textbf{O}_1 \quad \textbf{X} \quad \textbf{O}_2$$

FIGURE 2 One-group pretest-posttest design.

If the staff satisfaction study we just mentioned had included a pretest, it would have had a design like the one shown in Figure 2. Similar to the One-Shot Case Study, this design lacks a control group, which prevents the researcher from making the causal inference that the observed value of the dependent variable is due to the independent variable, instead of *history, maturation,* or even *testing.* This design is now known as a "single group study" or a "single arm study," which is the aforementioned design in the hypothetical study described by Taylor and Asmundson (2008), in which *maturation* (disease progression) was confounded with the independent variable (an antidepressant medication), such that the researchers mistakenly concluded that the improved mood of the study participants was due to the antidepressants.

Despite its severe limitations, this design has gained acceptance in certain areas of healthcare research (Ip et al., 2013), especially quality improvement studies (McLaughlin & Kaluzny, 2006; Van Bokhoven, Kok, & Van der Weijden, 2003). However, the Agency for Healthcare Research and Quality of the U.S. Department of Health and Human Services has said it is not appropriate for assessing the effectiveness of clinical interventions (Ip et al., 2013).

If the study participants were selected for a One-Shot Case Study because of their high or low scores, *regression toward the mean* would also pose a threat to internal validity. However, this problem could be remedied by adding a second pretest: $O_1 \ O_2 \ \mathbf{X} \ O_3$. The researcher would then compare the values of the dependent variable at O_2 and O_3 to assess the effect of the independent variable $\mathbf{X}$, because *regression toward the mean* should have occurred between O_1 and O_2.

JHCC has published three articles that used the design in Figure 2, which is probably the most common design used in program evaluation studies. The three studies provide valuable information about the usefulness of their programs (i.e., their independent variables) without making claims regarding the effectiveness of the independent variables. The first article reported that a workshop on pastoral-care research improved "chaplains" feelings and attitudes regarding research (Murphy & Fitchett, 2009). The second article reported that a chaplain-led spiritual intervention with community-dwelling older adults improved their sense of connection to others and feelings about life, including a sense of gratitude (Grewe, 2017), and the third article reported that a chaplain-led spiritual intervention with U.S. Veterans Administration patients reduced their sense of spiritual distress (Kopacz, Adams, & Searle, 2017).

Static Group Comparison

Campbell (1957) called the third pre-experimental design, the Static Group Comparison, which is shown in Figure 3. Cook and Campbell (1979) later

Group 1   X   O

Group 2   O

FIGURE 3 Static group comparison.

called this a Posttest-Only Design with Nonequivalent Groups. Unlike the first two designs we have discussed, this design consists of two groups: Group 1 receives an intervention before the dependent variable is measured, whereas Group 2 does not receive the intervention.

A researcher might be inclined to use this design to compare the effects of a medical intervention with patients on one hospital unit to the effects of standard care with patients on another hospital unit, but this would be a bad idea, as this design fails to control for *history, maturation,* and *selection bias; selection bias* is always a threat to internal validity unless participants are randomly assigned to the study groups. Nevertheless, this is the basic design used in epidemiological case-control studies, with **X** representing exposure to some disease-promoting agent or event, also known as a risk factor (Kelsey, Thompson, & Evans, 1986; Kleinbaum, Kupper, & Morgenstern, 1982). A common way for epidemiologists to attempt to control for *history* is to match the individuals they select for the unexposed group (the "control," or more appropriately the "comparison" group) with the exposed group as best as they can on different variables, such as profession, type of work, neighborhood, or workplace, depending on the type of exposure being investigated (Kleinbaum et al., 1982). *Maturation* in the most general sense can be achieved by matching for age and gender. Other approaches to selecting a "control" or "comparison" group is to draw random samples from: (a) the general population that appears to be the same as the case population, (b) neighborhoods similar to those where the cases live, and (c) persons seeking medical care at the same hospitals where the cases sought care (Kelsey et al., 1986).

INTERNAL VALIDITY OF THREE EXPERIMENTAL DESIGNS

All true experimental designs entail random assignment of the study's participants to the experimental and control groups at the start of the experiment, which is indicated by **R** in Figures 4–6. Random assignment can be conducted in many ways, including something as simple as flipping a coin if there are only two groups: heads = experimental group, tails = control group, or vice versa.

Posttest-Only Control Group Design

The experimental design Campbell (1957) called the Posttest-Only Control Group Design, which is depicted in Figure 4, is identical to the

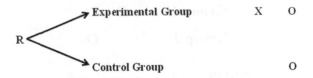

FIGURE 4 Posttest-only control group design.

pre-experimental design that Campbell called the One-Shot Case Study, depicted in Figure 1, except that the Posttest-Only Control Group Design includes the random assignment of participants to groups or conditions (i.e., the experimental condition and control condition). As previously mentioned, *selection bias* is the threat that the participants assigned to the experimental and control groups are not equivalent. Random assignment to groups is used to eliminate the threat of *selection bias* and thereby ensure that the experimental and control groups are equivalent at the start of the experiment.

Although Campbell and Stanley (1966) simply inserted an **R** before each group to indicate random assignment to groups, we think Figure 4 provides a better depiction of random assignment, because it illustrates that the participants are randomly assigned from a common pool of participants who will serve in either the experimental or the control group.

The Posttest-Only Control Group Design is one of the most widely used designs in animal research, especially physiological and behavioral studies on "laboratory" rats and mice. Many animal studies do not require a pretest of the dependent variable because the previous experience of the animals is carefully controlled to make them similar, or more technically, to minimize the variation between the animals: their experience is controlled by the temperature and light/dark cycle of the rooms they live in, the standardized cages they live in, the food they eat, their feeding schedules, and so forth. This greatly reduces the likelihood that they will differ on the dependent variable at the start of an experiment; hence, a pretest of the dependent variable is usually not deemed necessary. Inclusion and exclusion criteria in human medical research also makes it possible to use this design in RCTs because the criteria create a relatively homogeneous pool of participants who are then assigned to the experimental and control groups (Salmond, 2008). This is a worthwhile design for RCTs of the effects of an independent variable on physical/physiological outcomes (i.e., dependent variables), but it is not recommended for studies of psychological outcomes, which usually employ a pretest to measure the dependent variable before the independent variable is introduced.

The remaining threats to the internal validity of such studies, like all studies, are *history* and *maturation,* which are controlled in this design by having a control group (also called the untreated group) that is compared to the experimental group (also called the treated group). The effects of the treatment or intervention are statistically analyzed simply by comparing the data on the dependent variable from the two groups at point **O**. This analysis can easily be performed with a *t*-test if the data are suitable for such an analysis, in terms of the level of measurement with which the dependent variable is measured [see *JHCC* articles by Jankowski, Flannelly, & Flannelly (2017) regarding *t*-tests, and L. T. Flannelly et al. (2014b) regarding levels of measurement]. A *t*-test is appropriate for analyzing data measured on an interval or ratio scale.

Pretest–Posttest Control Group Design

Because humans vary in many ways, researchers usually want to demonstrate the equivalence of the experimental and control groups before an experiment by conducting a pretest (de Boer, Waterlander, Kuijper, Steenhuis, & Twisk, 2015), as shown in Figure 5. In addition to pretesting the dependent variable, pretests in healthcare studies typically measure the personal characteristics of participants (e.g., socio-demographic variables, general indices of physical mental and health) to see if the experimental and control groups differ in other ways—aside from the dependent variable—that might affect the outcome of the experiment.

This design is the solution to the aforementioned problem posed in the hypothetical study in which the effect of *maturation* (progression of Alzheimer's disease) on depression was mistakenly thought be the effect of antidepressant medication. The control group in this design not only controls for the possible effects of *maturation,* it also controls for the effects of *history, regression toward the mean,* and *instrumentation* on the dependent variable. This design is widely used as a two-arm RCT.

Of course, the experimental and control arms must be conducted during the same period of time, as shown in the diagram. The control arm cannot be conducted after the experimental arm, as it was in our hypothetical example of an experiment on the effectiveness of a family program to reduce childhood obesity. One should think of a large study that is conducted over time as a series of smaller studies consisting of cohorts of experimental and control participants and be aware that threats to internal validity have to be addressed for each cohort. The cohort could be as small as two; that is, whenever two individuals consent to participate in a study, one could be randomly assigned to the experimental group and one to the control group.

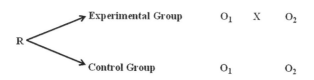

FIGURE 5 Pretest-posttest control group design.

Random assignment to groups controls for *selection bias* in this design, as it did in the Posttest-Only Control Group Design. As *selection bias* is a potential bias when assigning participants to experimental and control groups, the use of inclusion and exclusion criteria can decrease the threat of *selection bias* because they decrease individual differences within the pool of participants on variables that are likely to affect the dependent variable. However, as Campbell (1957) discussed, the homogeneity of the pool of participants that these criteria create reduces the external validity (i.e., the generalizability) of a study's results.

The possible effect of *mortality* can initially be assessed by comparing the *drop-out rates* of the two groups at the end of the study. If the *drop-out rates* are comparable, there is no reason to believe that *mortality* is a threat to the experiment's internal validity. More extensive comparisons of the information collected on the experimental and control participants during the pretest need to be performed if the *drop-out rates* differ substantially between the groups. Although this design controls for *regression toward the mean* because both groups are given a pretest and a posttest, the use of a pretest introduces the threat of a *testing* effect that cannot be isolated with this design.

Campbell recommended statistically analyzing the effects of the independent variable on the dependent variable in this design by calculating difference scores (posttest - pretest) for each participant and comparing the average difference score (also called a change score) of the two groups using a *t*-test. Campbell and Stanley (1966) recommended that the analysis of the difference scores should statistically control for participants' pretest scores by using them as a covariate in the analysis, which requires using a statistical procedure called analysis of covariance (ANCOVA). Although a discussion of ANCOVA lies outside the scope of this article, the analysis recommended by Campbell and Stanley is the preferred way to analyze these data (Takona, 2002) [see Keppel & Wickens (2004), Tabachnick & Fidell, 2013 or a similar book for a description of ANCOVA]. Similar to the *t*-test, ANCOVA is only appropriate for analyzing interval or ratio data.

Naturally, the longer the time-span is between the pretest and the posttest, the greater the likelihood is that *history* and *maturation* will pose a threat to the internal validity of an experiment. Therefore, pretests and posttests should be administered as close to the beginning and end of the intervention as possible. However, a researcher may want to assess the long-term effects of the independent variable on the dependent variable. This can be assessed by adding another posttest (O_3) at some point in time after the initial posttest (O_2) to both groups in Figure 5, which would be shown as O_2 O_3. These data can also be analyzed to statistically control for participants' pretest scores (O_1) using ANCOVA if all the data are interval or ratio variables (Twisk & de Vente, 2008). A statistical procedure called logistic regression is often used to control for pretest scores when the dependent variable is dichotomous or binomial, such as "case/no-case" (Kleinbaum, Kupper, Nizam, & Rosenberm, 2014).

Solomon Four-Group Design

This design, which is shown in Figure 6, controls for all seven threats to internal validity: *history, maturation, instrumentation, regression toward the mean, selection, mortality,* and *testing*. However, it does not appear to be widely used in healthcare research. This is probably because it is time-consuming and costly to run four groups of participants just to control for the effects of *testing*, especially as: (a) the Pretest-Posttest Control Group Design controls for all of the threats to internal validity except *testing,* and (b) there may be no reason for the researcher to believe the tests used to measure the dependent variable are reactive measures.

Nevertheless, we will explain it briefly. The four groups in the design are created by randomly assigning participants to each group, which controls for *selection bias.* The design is obviously a combination of the designs illustrated in Figures 4 and 5. While Group 1 measures changes due to the independent variable, Group 2 controls for the effects of *history* and *maturation,* which always offer competing explanations for the apparent effect of the independent variable ($\mathbf{X}$) on the dependent variable ($\mathbf{O}$). Group 2 also controls for the possible confounds of *regression toward the mean* and *instrumentation.*

Since Groups 3 and 4 do not include pretests, they control for the effects of *testing* (the pretest) on the posttest scores of the dependent variable in Groups 1 and 2, respectively. Campbell recommends the 2×2 analysis of variance (ANOVA) shown in Figure 7 to analyze the effects of *testing* on the final (right-hand) measures ($\mathbf{O}$'s) of the dependent variable shown in Figure 6. This diagram implies that the analysis assesses the main effect of pretest (Yes or No), the main effect of treatment ($\mathbf{X}=$ Yes or No) and the interaction of pretest and treatment [see Keppel & Wickens (2004) or a similar book for a description of ANOVA].

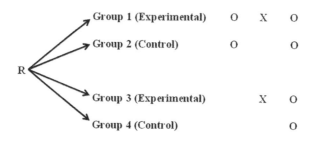

FIGURE 6 Solomon four-group design.

	X = Yes	X = No
Pretest = Yes	Group 1	Group 2
Pretest = No	Group 3	Group 4

FIGURE 7 ANOVA to assess the effect of *testing* in the Solomon four-group design.

INTERNAL VALIDITY OF SELECTED QUASI-EXPERIMENTAL DESIGNS

Nonequivalent Control Group Design

Campbell and Stanley (1966) said this was the most frequently used design in educational research and it seems that it still is (Takona, 2002). The design, which is shown in Figure 8, consists of two groups: one that receives an intervention (the independent variable) at point **X** and one that does not. A pretest (O_1) and posttest (O_2) is given to each group. The **A** indicates that the study participants are assigned to each group, but the assignment is not randomized (Campbell & Stanley, 1966). Cook and Campbell (1979), who said it was the most frequently used design in social science research, gave it the unwieldy name, "The Untreated Control Group Design with Pretest and Posttest."

Typically, entire classes of students are assigned to groups in educational research, instead of assigning individual students to groups, which makes the design easy to implement in educational settings. However, the design is subject to *selection bias* because of the lack of random assignment to groups. As an example, students in different classes that are grouped by ability (also known as academic tracking) could cause *selection bias*. Although this would be an obvious problem that a researcher could easily avoid by selecting two classes at the same academic level, the composition of classes might differ for reasons that could be far less obvious to a researcher. As the experimental and control groups are not equivalent because participants are not randomly assigned to groups, the "control" group in this design is usually called a "comparison" group.

This design also applies to the previously described hypothetical study of quality of life of patients undergoing HD, in which the researcher assigned the patients to the experimental and control groups based on the days of the week they attended the HD center (MWF vs. TTS). As previously noted, there may be many reasons why the patients chose to receive HD on MWF

A	Experimental Group	O_1	X	O_2
A	Control Group	O_1		O_2

FIGURE 8 Nonequivalent control group design.

vs. TTS, and their reasons could affect the study's outcomes. One reason could be that some patients may choose MWF for convenience because they do not work and they want their weekends free, whereas other patients may choose TTS because they work and they cannot take three weekdays off from their jobs. Another reason might be that relatives and friends drive the patient to and from the HD center, and one of them is only available to do so on weekends.

Like the Pretest–Posttest Control Group Design shown in Figure 5, this design controls for *maturation,* and, to some extent, it controls for *history,* although the experiences of participants may differ somewhat on MWF than TTS. However, we came across a quasi-experimental study comparing the effects of standard care and patient-centered care after hip surgery, which might appear to be a Nonequivalent Control Group Design, but obviously does not control for *history* (Olsson, Karlsson, Berg, Kärrholm, & Hansson, 2014). That study did not control for *history* because the experimental condition (the patients who received patient-centered care) was conducted nine months after the control condition (the patients who received standard care) was conducted, and the control and experimental conditions (or groups) have to be conducted during the same time-period to control for *history.*

An actual Nonequivalent Control Group Design also controls for the effects of *regression toward the mean,* and *instrumentation* on the dependent variable. Once again, potential differences in *drop-out rates* pose the threat of *mortality.* As previously mentioned, however, if the *drop-out rates* are similar, there is no reason to believe that *mortality* is a threat to the study's internal validity. Because this study employs a pretest and a posttest, it is possible that *testing* poses a threat to its internal validity.

Similar to the Pretest–Posttest Control Group Design, the best way to analyze the data is to perform ANCOVA on the posttest–pretest change scores, using the pretest score as a covariate. Although the design does not control for *selection bias,* if the pretest included measures of variables that might be expected to affect the dependent variable, they can also be used as covariates in the ANCOVA. For example, in the study on the quality of life of HD patients, it would be valuable to measure employment and social support during the pretest, and, therefore, they can be controlled for statistically in the analysis of changes in quality of life.

Pretest–Posttest Two Treatment Group Design

Figure 9 illustrates a design, which we named a Pretest-Posttest Two Treatment Group Design. The design has the same flaws and most of the benefits of the Pretest-Posttest Control Group Design, but one cannot be sure the changes observed over time in either group would not have occurred without any treatment. Yet, this design can be useful for comparing different treatment or intervention effects. This is the basic design used by Jankowski,

A	Experimental Group A	O_1	X_A	O_2
A	Experimental Group B	O_1	X_B	O_2

FIGURE 9 Pretest-posttest two treatment group design.

Vanderwerker, Murphy, Montonye, and Ross (2008) to compare changes in pastoral skills, self-reflection, and other variables in clinical pastoral care (CPE) students who took a short/intensive CPE course (X_A) or a long-extended CPE course (X_B).

The length of the intervention (the CPE course) differed, suggesting that the confounding effect of *history* is problematic for the study's internal validity. *Selection bias* is another serious threat to the study's internal validity because the students chose which course they would take. Jankowski et al. (2008) tried to address this threat (a) by obtaining pretest measures of age, gender, years in ministry, years of theological education, and prior CPE training; and (b) using multiple regression to statistically control for the effects of these variables on the change scores of the dependent variables (simple regression is discussed by Flannelly, Flannelly, & Jankowski, 2016).

Cook and Campbell (1979) described a similar design with two treatment groups that they called "The Reversed-Treatment Nonequivalent Control Group Design with Pretest and Posttest." As the name implies, the two independent variables in such a study are designed to produce reverse or opposite effects on the dependent variable. If the opposite directional effects are observed at the posttest, this makes a logically compelling case that the observed effects are due to the independent variables, even though it lacks a control group that does not receive either treatment.

Time-Series Designs

Campbell and Stanley (1966) illustrated several time-series designs, the first of which they simply called **The Time Series Experiment**. This design is particularly useful when there is a system for collecting data on some variable of interest (i.e., the dependent variable) across an extended period of time on a regular periodic schedule. Figure 10 shows a time-series experiment in which the dependent variable is measured each month for 12 months, with the intervention introduced about the sixth month of data collection. The design provides evidence for the effect of the independent variable on the dependent variable, if the introduction of the independent variable (X) alters the dependent variable.

$$O_1 \quad O_2 \quad O_3 \quad O_4 \quad O_5 \quad O_6 \ X \ O_7 \quad O_8 \quad O_9 \quad O_{10} \quad O_{11} \quad O_{12}$$

FIGURE 10 The time series experiment.

To make the discussion more concrete, assume that a hospital system wanted to conduct a study to evaluate the effectiveness of a pilot program to increase the use of advance directives before investing in a full program. This design would be a reasonable choice because it controls for *testing, regression toward the mean, maturation,* and *mortality*. It controls for *testing* because the measurement of the dependent variable is nonreactive, as it would be the regular monthly summary of the number of patients who signed advance directives. It controls *regression toward the mean* because extreme values in either direction that are due to chance would balance out across the time series. It mainly controls for *maturation* and *mortality* because most of the patients without advance directives are unique patients at each time-point. Campbell and Stanley (1966) said the design controls for *selection bias,* but it fails to control for *instrumentation* and *history*.

The preferred design for this study is shown in Figure 11, which Campbell and Stanley (1966) called The Multiple Time Series Design. A hospital system could easily employ this design, because it could introduce an intervention in one of its hospitals and use another hospital as a control or comparison. If the intervention (**X**) continues over time past O_7, the design would be depicted as a series of **X**'s between O_7 and O_{12}.

The design controls for everything that the design in Figure 10 does and more. Most importantly, it controls for *history*. The most obvious reasons why *history* might pose a threat to the study's internal validity are public efforts to promote the use of advance directives or the recent hospitalization of a family member or friend with a fatal illness who did not have the capacity to make their own health care decisions. It controls for *instrumentation* because the definition of what advanced directives would not be expected to change over time in both hospitals.

There are several ways to analyze both of these designs. With six observations before and after the intervention, one could conduct a single-sample *t*-test on the mean number of pre- and postintervention advance directives in the first design. The analysis of the means should be conducted in the multiple time-series design using ANOVA. It would probably be worthwhile to measure the dependent variable for all the analyses as the percentage of new advance directives by patients who did not initially have them.

Another way to analyze the effect of the independent variable on the dependent variable is to conduct separate regression analyses on the pre- and post-intervention data and statistically compare the slopes of their trend lines. If the dependent variable is measured as a percentage or other

O_1 O_2 O_3 O_4 O_5 O_6 X O_7 O_8 O_9 O_{10} O_{11} O_{12}

O_1 O_2 O_3 O_4 O_5 O_6 O_7 O_8 O_9 O_{10} O_{11} O_{12}

FIGURE 11 The multiple time series design.

proportion, one could also use the Change-Point Test to assess whether the independent variable affected the dependent variable (Siegel & Castellan, 1988).

Summary

Of the seven threats to the internal validity of an experiment that we discussed, *history* and *maturation* should be thought of as universal threats because they are always present when an independent variable is present. More sophisticated experimental designs tend to introduce new threats to internal validity that must be controlled as they attempt to eliminate other threats. These threats include *testing, instrument decay, regression toward the mean, selection,* and *mortality.* All seven threats to internal validity are problematic because they offer alternate explanations for the observed effects of an experiment on the dependent variable, other than the independent variable. Therefore, it is imperative that researchers understand these threats as they apply to any experimental design chosen and implemented by a researcher. Science moves forward only as far as good research design permits.

Finally, although we only mentioned inclusion and exclusion criteria in passing, we noted that they are useful in health care research to create a relatively homogeneous pool of participants who can be assigned to the experimental and control groups. While the homogeneity of a sample is useful for assessing the experimental effects of an independent variable on a dependent variable, it reduces the external validity (i.e., the generalizability) of the experimental findings (Campbell, 1957).

NOTES

1. The term "single-arm study" is explained later in the article.
2. We do not know if the blood-pressure readings actually decrease when the battery is low, but this is a hypothetical example.
3. The Karnofsky Performance Scale ranges from $0 =$ Dead to $100 =$ Normal, no complaints, no evidence of disease. Some other points on the scale include: $20 =$ Very sick, hospital admission necessary, active supportive treatment necessary; $40 =$ Disabled, requires special care and assistance; $60 =$ Requires occasional assistance, but is able to care for most of his/her personal needs; and $80 =$ Normal activity with effort, some signs or symptoms or disease.

REFERENCES

Bernard, C. (1865/1957). *An introduction to the study of experimental medicine.* New York, NY: Dover.

Campbell, D. T. (1957). Factors relevant to the validity of experiments in social settings. *Psychological Bulletin, 54*(4), 297–312. doi:10.1037/h0040950

Campbell, D. T., & Stanley, J. C. (1966). *Experimental and quasi-experimental designs for research.* Chicago, IL: Rand McNally & Company.

Cherulnik, P. D. (1983). *Behavioral research: Assessing the validity of research findings in psychology.* Philadelphia, PA: Harper & Row.

Cook, T. D., & Campbell, D. T. (1979). *Quasi-experimentation: Design & analysis issues for field settings.* Boston, MA: Houghton Mifflin.

Crooks, V., Waller, S., Smith, T., & Hahn, T. J. (1991). The use of the Karnofsky Performance Scale in determining outcomes and risk in geriatric outpatients. *Journal of Gerontology, 46*(4), M139–M144. doi:10.1093/geronj/46.4.m139

de Boer, M. R., Waterlander, W. E., Kuijper, L. D., Steenhuis, I. H., & Twisk, J. W. (2015). Testing for baseline differences in randomized controlled trials: An unhealthy research behavior that is hard to eradicate. *International Journal of Behavioral Nutrition and Physical Activity, 12*(1), 4. doi:10.1186/s12966-015-0162-z

Derrickson, P., & Van Hise, A. (2010). Curriculum for a spiritual pathway project: Integrating research methodology into pastoral care training. *Journal of Health Care Chaplaincy, 16*(1–2), 3–12. doi:10.1080/08854720903451030

Flannelly, K. J., Flannelly, L. T., & Jankowski, K. R. B. (2016). Studying associations in health care research. *Journal of Health Care Chaplaincy, 22*(3), 118–131. doi:10.1080/08854726.2016.1194046

Flannelly, K. J., & Jankowski, K. R. B. (2014). Research designs and making causal inferences from healthcare studies. *Journal of Health Care Chaplaincy, 20*(1), 23–38. doi:10.1080/08854726.2014.871909

Flannelly, L. T., Flannelly, K. J., & Jankowski, K. R. B. (2014a). Independent, dependent, and other variables in healthcare and chaplaincy research. *Journal of Health Care Chaplaincy, 20*(4), 161–170. doi:10.1080/08854726.2014.959374

Flannelly, L. T., Flannelly, K. J., & Jankowski, K. R. B. (2014b). Fundamentals of measurement in healthcare research. *Journal of Health Care Chaplaincy, 20*(2), 75–82. doi:10.1080/08854726.2014.906262

Fleenor, D., Sharma, V., Hirschmann, J., & Swarts, H. (2017). Do journal clubs work? The effectiveness of journal clubs in a clinical pastoral education residency program. *Journal of Health Care Chaplaincy*, 1–14. doi:10.1080/08854726.2017.1383646

Greenhalgh, T. (2001). *How to read a paper: The basics of evidence based medicine.* London, UK: BMJ Books.

Grewe, F. (2017). The Soul's Legacy: A program designed to help prepare senior adults cope with end-of-life existential distress. *Journal of Health Care Chaplaincy, 23*(1), 1–14. doi:10.1080/08854726.2016.1194063

Ip, S., Paulus, J. K., Balk, E. M., Dahabreh, I. J., Avendano, E. E., & Lau, J (2013). Role of single group studies in Agency for Healthcare Research and Quality comparative effectiveness reviews. Research white paper (Prepared by Tufts Evidence-based Practice Center under Contract No. 290–2007-10055-I) (AHRQ Publication No. 13-EHC007-EF). Rockville, MD: Agency for Healthcare Research and Quality. Retrieved from www.effectivehealthcare.ahrq.gov

Jackson-Jordan, E., Stafford, C., Stratton, S. V., Vilagos, T. T., Janssen Keenan, A., & Greg Hathaway, G. (2017). Evaluation of a chaplain residency program and its partnership with an in-patient palliative care team. *Journal of Health Care Chaplaincy*, 1–10. doi:10.1080/08854726.2017.1324088

Jankowski, K. R., Vanderwerker, L. C., Murphy, K. M., Montonye, M., & Ross, A. M. (2008). Change in pastoral skills, emotional intelligence, self-reflection, and social desirability across a unit of CPE. *Journal of Health Care Chaplaincy,* *15*(2), 132–148. doi:10.1080/08854720903163304

Jankowski, K. R. B., Flannelly, K. J., & Flannelly, L. T. (2017). The *t*-test: An influential inferential tool in chaplaincy and other healthcare research. *Journal of Health Care Chaplaincy,* 1–10. doi:10.1080/08854726.2017.1335050

Kane, R. L. (Ed.). (2005). *Understanding health care outcomes research* (2nd ed.). Sudbury, MA: Jones & Bartlett.

Keele, R. (2012). *Nursing research and evidence-based practice: Ten steps to success.* Sudbury, MA: Jones & Bartlett Learning.

Kelsey, J., Thompson, W. D., & Evans, A. S. (1986). *Methods in observational epidemiology.* New York, NY: Oxford University Press.

Keppel, G. & Wickens, T. D. (2004). *Design and analysis: A researcher's handbook* (4th ed.). Upper Saddle River, NJ: Pearson Prentice Hall.

Kerlinger, F. N. (1973). *Foundations of behavioral research* (2nd ed.). New York, NY: Holt, Rinehart, and Winston.

Kleinbaum, D. G., Kupper, L. L., & Morgenstern, H. (1982). *Epidemiolic research: Principles and quantitative methods.* New York, NY: Van Nostrand Reinhold.

Kleinbaum, D. G., Kupper, L. L., Nizam, A., & Rosenberm E. S. (2014). *Applied regression analysis and other multivariable methods* (5th ed.). Boston MA: Cengage Learning.

Kopacz, M. S., Adams, M. S., & Searle, R. F. (2017). Lectio Divina: A preliminary evaluation of a chaplaincy program. *Journal of Health Care Chaplaincy,* *23*(3), 87–97. doi:10.1080/08854726.2016.1253263

Lennon-Dearing, R., Florence, J. A., Halvorson, H., & Pollard, J. T. (2012). An interprofessional educational approach to teaching spiritual assessment. *Journal of Health Care Chaplaincy,* *18*(3–4), 121–132. doi:10.1080/ 08854726.2012.720546

McLaughlin, C. P., & Kaluzny, A. D. (2006). *Continuous quality improvement in health care: Theories, implementations, and applications* (3rd ed.). Sudbury MA: Jones and Bartlett.

Mill, J. S. (1859). *A system of logic, ratiocinative and inductive; bring a connected view of the principles of evidence and the methods of scientific investigation.* New York, NY: Harper & Brothers.

Murphy, P. E., & Fitchett, G. (2009). Introducing chaplains to research: "This could help me." *Journal of Health Care Chaplaincy,* *16*(3–4), 79–94. doi:10.1080/ 08854726.2010.480840

Olsson, L. E., Karlsson, J., Berg, U., Kärrholm, J., & Hansson, E. (2014). Person-centred care compared with standardized care for patients undergoing total hip arthroplasty—A quasi-experimental study. *Journal of Orthopaedic Surgery and Research,* *9*(1), 95. doi:10.1186/s13018-014-0095-2

Rubinson, L., & Neutens, J. J. (1987). *Research techniques for the health sciences.* New York, NY: Macmillan Publishing.

Salmond, S. S. (2008). Randomized controlled trials: Methodological concepts and critique. *Orthopaedic Nursing,* *27*(2), 116–122. doi:10.1097/01.nor. 0000315626.44137.94

Siegel, S., & Castellan, N. J. (1988). *Nonparametric statistics for the behavioral sciences* (2nd ed.). New York, NY: McGraw-Hill.

Tabachnick, B. G., & Fidell, L. S. (2013). *Using multivariate statistics* (6th ed.). Boston, MA: Pearson.

Takona, J. P. (2002). *Educational research: Principles and practice*. Lincoln, NE: Writers Club Press.

Tappan, R. M. (2015). *Advanced nursing research* (2nd ed.) Sudbury, MA: Jones & Bartlett Learning.

Taylor, S., & Asmundson, G. J. G. (2008). Internal and external validity in clinical research. In D. McKay (Ed.), *Handbook of research methods in abnormal and clinical psychology* (pp. 23–34). Los Angeles, CA: Sage.

Terret, C., Albrand, G., Moncenix, G., & Droz, J. P. (2011). Karnofsky Performance Scale (KPS) or Physical Performance Test (PPT)? That is the question. *Critical Reviews in Oncology/Hematology*, *77*(2), 142–147. doi:10.1016/j.critrevonc. 2010.01.015

Twisk, J. W., & de Vente, W. (2008). The analysis of randomised controlled trial data with more than one follow-up measurement. A comparison between different approaches. *European Journal of Epidemiology*, *23*(10), 655–660. doi:10.1007/ s10654-008-9279-6

Van Bokhoven, M. A., Kok, G., & Van der Weijden, T. (2003). Designing a quality improvement intervention: A systematic approach. *Quality and Safety in Health Care*, *12*(3), 215–220. doi:10.1136/qhc.12.3.215

Webb, E. J., Campbell, D. T., Schwartz, R. D., & Sechrest, L. (1966). *Unobtrusive measures: Nonreactive research in the social sciences*. Chicago, IL: Rand McNally.

Index

Note: Page numbers followed by italics and bold refers to figures and tables respectively.

101, 101–3; Solomon four-group design
103, *103*, *104*
experimental mortality *see* mortality, internal
validity of experiment
experimental research 8–10
experimentation 11
extraneous variable 38, 39

Fetzer Institutes scale 28, 29
Fisher, Ronald A. 79
Fitchett, G. 8
Flannelly, K. J. 41, 67
Flannelly, L. T. 41, 67
Framingham Heart Study 7, 38
frequency measures 41

Galton, F. 5–6
galvanic-skin-response (GSR) 93
Gaudette, H. 37
Gaussian distribution 61
Gay-Lussac, J. 65
Gibson, T. M. 76
Gosset, W. S. 79, 81
grade point average (GPA) 20
Grossoehme, D. H. 37
Guinness, C. 79

Handbook of Religion and Health 29–30
Helgadóttir, H. L. 48
Hill, A. B. 71–3
Hill, P. C. 28
history, internal validity of experiment 91
Hofler, M. 73
Hood Jr., R. W. 28
Hungler, B. P. 20
hypertension 40
hypothetical anxiety scores *51*, 51–2
hypothetical distributions of pain ratings **56**,
56–8, *57*
hypothetical scale 56

independent variable and dependent variable
35–6; categorical 41; confounding 38–9;
continuous 41; discrete 41; extraneous
38, 39; intervening 39; mediating 39;
moderating 40–1; nuisance 38; outcomes
37; predictor 37; protective factor 38;
response 37; risk factor 38; statistical
analyses 39; treatment and intervention
36–7
instrument decay, internal validity of
experiment 93–4
internal validity of experiments: experimental
designs *see* experimental designs, internal
validity; pre-experimental designs
see pre-experimental designs, internal
validity; quasi-experimental design

see quasi-experimental design, internal
validity; threats to *see* threats to internal
validity of experiments
International Statistical Classification of
Diseases and Related Health Problems
(ICD) 29
interpretation of t-test 84
interquartile range (IQR) 58
interval measurement 21–2
intervening variable 39
intervention and treatment 36–7

Jankowski, K. R. B. 37, 41, 67, 105–6
Joint Method of Agreement and Difference
(Mill) 9
Journal of Health Care Chaplaincy (JHCC)
1–2, 5, 6, 8, 11, 19, 36, 55–6, 67, 69, 81, 82,
97, 98

Kerlinger, F. N. 1
Kerlinger, Fred 96–7
Kleinbaum, D. G. 73
Koenig, H. G. 29

large-scale descriptive studies 5
La Touche, Christopher 79
Levin, J. S. 26–7, 40
Life and Labour of the People of London 5
linear associations 77
linear regression 68
linear relationships 69
The Logic of Logic on Modern Physics
(Bridgman) 25
longitudinal study 12

McPhail, G. L. 37
Markman, M. 36
mathematical formulas 65
maturation, internal validity of experiment
91–2
mean 50–2, *51*
measurement: interval 21–2; nominal 18–19;
ordinal 19–21; ratio 22–3; value of 23; *see
also* central tendency measure; variability
measure
median 46–50, **47**, *49*
mediating variable 39
Medical Outcomes Study 36-Item Short-Form
Health Survey (SF-36) 30–1, 48
mental disorders, operational definitions
29–30
Method of Concomitant Variations (Mill) 8, 9
Methods of Residues (Mill) 8
Mill, J. S. 8–9, 11, 71, 72
mode 45–6
moderating variable 40–1
Montonye, M. 37, 105–6

For Product Safety Concerns and Information please contact our EU
representative GPSR@taylorandfrancis.com Taylor & Francis Verlag GmbH,
Kaufingerstraße 24, 80331 München, Germany

Printed and bound by CPI Group (UK) Ltd, Croydon, CR0 4YY

08/06/2025

01896991-0018